BLACK MEDICINE VOL. II
Weapons At Hand

by
N. Mashiro, Ph.D.

Black Medicine Vol. II
Weapons at Hand
by N. Mashiro, Ph.D.
Copyright © 1979 by Paladin Press

ISBN 0-87364-168-X
Printed in the United States of America

Published by Paladin Press, a division of
Paladin Enterprises, Inc., P.O. Box 1307,
Boulder, Colorado 80306, USA.
(303) 443-7250

Direct inquiries and/or orders to the above address.

Library of Congress Cataloging in Publication Data:
Mashiro, N.
    Black Medicine, Vol. II, Weapons at Hand

    1. Hand-to-hand fighting   2. Hand-to-hand fighting, Oriental
3. Self-defense.   I. Title.
GV1111.M359   613.6'6   79-2210

TABLE OF CONTENTS

INTRODUCTION

The first volume of this series (**Black Medicine: The Dark Art of Death**) discussed over 150 parts of the human body which are especially vulnerable in hand-to-hand combat. The present volume is a direct outgrowth of the previous one. **Black Medicine Vol. II: Weapons at Hand** presents 112 parts of the body which are natural weapons, largely because they are very resistant to injury. Even if stripped naked and bound securely a resourceful combat artist can still bring many of these natural weapons into play to the detriment of this tormentors. In this sense the body's natural weapons constitute *weapons at hand.*

The second half of this book contains suggestions toward a new art of makeshift weaponry. In it are listed over 180 common makeshift weapons which may be available in a crisis. The orientation of this discussion is especially appropriate to the victim of a kidnapping, a hostage held by terrorists or a prisoner of war. Any person who is disarmed and desperate will appreciate the information in this volume, especially since most terrorist kidnap victims are killed, not rescued or ransomed. Saving the life of the victim is usually a do-it-yourself proposition.

It is traditional in books about self-defense for the author to make allusions to the rising crime rate and the fact that the streets of America are dangerous. Usually there is some comment like "just glance through the newspaper to see how often violent confrontations really occur." Self-defense authors write such comments because they have to justify their obvious preoccupation with violence. Many people seem to think that the authors of books such as this one are mentally unbalanced. We get sensitive about it. I think the main difference between martial artists and "normal" people is that we martial artists

1

have managed to overcome the widespread head-in-the-sand syndrome. Violent events happen to all of us with surprising frequency, but most people prefer to ignore this unpleasant fact. To justify this statement, and to explain my personal interest in the combat arts, I have collected a few short horror stories which illustrate the point that violence really does surround us. All of these anecdotes are true, and all happened *to me or to people I know personally.*

1. We'll start with something simple. I have distinct childhood memories of playground bullies who terrorized smaller and less aggressive children. I was such a victim at one time. To adults this kind of thing seems mildly amusing in retrospect, but to the kids it is terrifying and very real. There are two points to make here. The first is that today's schools with their forced mixing of children from extremely different backgrounds are much more dangerous than the schools you and I attended. The bullies who pushed us around with their fists carry knives and guns now. Second, those playground terrorists often don't grow out of their perverse pleasure in causing other people pain. They become adults who delight in rearranging people's faces. Sooner or later we all meet one again.

2. A young man I work with was riding his $400 bicycle home after work one afternoon along a busy, well-traveled street in a fairly nice downtown area. Suddenly three black teenagers on bikes overtook him and started trying to force him into the curb. They were trying to steal the bicycle right out from under him! They didn't succeed, partly because the victim resisted their bungling attempts to spill him, and partly because four Chicanos pulled up in a car and joined the fray. The newcomers had clubs and made short work of scattering the blacks. Unfortunately they weren't rescuers. They wanted the bike for themselves. They got it.

3. My wife was discussing the above story with several ladies where she works. It turned out that my wife was the only woman in the room who had never been assaulted on the street. That revelation was very unsettling to her.

4. I knew a little old gentleman (about 5'4" tall and 65 years old) who routinely took his young puppy for a walk every

day. Master and puppy were taking care of their business one afternoon when three tough-looking teenagers walked up and demanded money. They made it clear that they were willing to beat the old gentleman into submission if he resisted. One of them demonstrated his contempt for life by viciously kicking the puppy. In most cases this situation would have ended in a successful robbery or mugging, but these unfortunate boys had selected the wrong little old man. He was a professional wrestling and self-defense coach. He knocked one of the thugs out cold and broke the leg of the second one. The third one proved that age does tell, however. He outran the enraged victim and got away.

5. My next door neighbor was driving home from work one night when he saw a young black couple with a gas can trying to flag him down. Being a generous Christian person he stopped and offered to give them a lift to a gas station. Once inside the car, the girl grabbed the wheel while the man clubbed my neighbor unconscious. He awakened several hours later, lying in an alley covered with his own blood. The hitch-hikers had obtained $25 from his wallet. He was very lucky that the blows to his head had produced only a mild concussion. The beating might easily have killed or crippled him.

6. Another neighbor was walking along the street when he encountered an angry teenage boy viciously beating a younger child. The neighbor intervened . . . and got a broken nose for his trouble.

7. A friend was walking home from work one night when he was accosted on the sidewalk by a robber carrying a .45 automatic. My friend was forced into an alley and relieved of his wallet and watch. Then the robber stepped closer, shoved the gun in my friend's stomach and fired. That might well have been the end of the story, but in this case the victim happened to be familiar both with firearms and with karate. When he saw the robber start to flinch in anticipation of the shot, my friend swatted the gun to the side. Then, before the second shot, he broke the neck of the would-be killer with a single blow.

8. My brother was visiting some hippie friends one time when a couple of nasty operators walked in and pulled out knives. They demanded cash, got it, and faded away into

3

the darkness. My brother's peace-loving friends looked like easy victims . . . and they were.

9. I once had a practice partner in a karate class who seemed very intent on causing me as much pain as possible. His tendency to strike with full power during periods when he was supposed to be holding back was extremely discourteous and disgraceful. Then he stopped coming to class. He had been arrested for armed robbery.

10. There was a period when I managed an apartment building and discovered one apartment full of deadbeat delinquents. They were the worst kind of vicious, drug-dulled dropouts. I had to evict them . . . personally. I read in the newspaper later that three of them are now in prison in connection with a murder-robbery.

11. One very significant episode occurred one evening when I was parking my car in front of my house. Just as I opened the door to get out a pickup truck came screeching around the corner and narrowly missed my open car door. Apparently the driver of the truck thought I had deliberately tried to cause an accident. He stopped his truck, jumped out, and came after me to teach me a lesson. It was fortunate, and somewhat amusing, that his wife collared him and dragged him back into the truck before he was able to carry out his intention. People who think they don't need self-defense because they avoid dangerous situations have not allowed for this kind of hot-headed person. All I did was to park in front of my own house.

12. Something similar happened to another close friend recently. He was driving to work in heavy traffic and made a lane change into a left-turn lane. For some reason this enraged the driver of the car behind him. The next thing my friend knew there was a very angry person trying to open his driver-side door. The door was locked. Frustrated, the assailant started banging on the window with a rock, trying to break in. That didn't work either. As a last resort this violent lunatic got back in his truck and deliberately rammed my friend's car. Then, satisfied, he drove away.

13. A former self-defense student of mine reported that he had been hitch-hiking along a country road when a girl picked him up and gave him a ride into town. When they arrived in town the student thanked the girl and got out of

her car. Just at that point a truck pulled up and a wild-eyed redneck leapt out. "I'll teach you to mess with my girl!" he shouted, and swung a roundhouse right at my student's face. My student had seen thousands of similar punches coming at him in my class, and he simply ducked. The furious attacker fell flat on his face. My student wisely left the scene.

14. I had another self-defense student who didn't have as much sense. He habitually frequented a bar where the resident yahoo delighted in wiping the floor with him. Every time he came to class he had new bruises. I mention this person to illustrate the fact that some victims are born and not made. Most of us know someone in this class.

15. Then there was the time I was driving home on the freeway after a pleasant evening at the theater. There was some night construction going on, and the freeway abruptly narrowed from four lanes to three. As traffic was merging into the remaining lanes a station wagon cut me off and stopped suddenly in front of me. I was not able to stop my car in time to avoid hitting it. Both cars pulled off to the shoulder. Then, like a bad dream, six black teenagers climbed out of the station wagon. All male and all mad. There were some bad moments before they decided to be civil. Confidence really shows in a situation like that.

16. My wife remembers vividly the time she walked out of a restaurant and found a man smashing windshields with a 2x4 in the parking lot. She watched helplessly as he moved down the line of cars breaking each windshield in turn, including hers. She was lucky that his animosity was directed only at cars.

17. Another time my wife was waiting at a stoplight when a strange man opened the passenger-side door and got in the car. After she ran a couple of red lights at seventy miles an hour he got out again . . . in a hurry.

18. I was once camping with a friend in a state park when I noticed a shadowy figure lurking in the gloom beyond the edge of the lantern light. I kept an eye out for him all evening, and eventually caught him sneaking up to the back of the tent. The police weren't interested. He was the local peeping tom and they knew that they couldn't convict him. The judge thought he was harmless.

19. On three occasions I have awakened in the middle of the

night and found a stranger prowling around in the backyard. This was at three different times, in three different backyards. Prowling must be fairly common.

20. My most vivid memory of the city of Denver has to do with a gas station in the downtown area. I pulled in for gas and couldn't get any attention from the employees. They were busy watching two mechanics slug it out with wrenches. Nobody was trying to stop the fight.

21. My grandfather had the unnerving experience of walking in on a burglary in progress in his own bedroom. He was lucky. The two young men ran instead of attacking him.

22. Speaking of burglaries, it's happened to me three times. There was also an incident in which my car was broken into by a thief in broad daylight.

23. A young friend was out bike riding one Saturday afternoon. She stopped at the side of the street to talk to a friend for a moment. As she was standing there holding her bicycle two men rode up on a motorcycle. One hopped off the motorcycle, knocked her down, and rode away on her bike. The two thieves were last seen threading their way through a crowed of pedestrians, none of whom would raise a hand to stop them.

24. I know a very gentle young woman who got into her car one day and found a man with a gun waiting for her. He had rape on his mind. He told her to drive him to a secluded spot he knew, but his plans went wrong. She started to cry and became so hysterical she couldn't control the car. He couldn't hold the gun and drive at the same time, so he gave up. Who says that crying doesn't help?

25. A neighbor lady answered her front door one morning to find a man with a gun, also intent on a rape/robbery. He was frustrated, too. She kicked him all the way down the front steps and chased him halfway down the block.

26. A third young female friend was the type who smiles at everybody. One day as she was walking down the street a tall black stranger engaged her in conversation. She was totally unequal to the situation. Getting raped is a terrible way to lose one's virginity, as she can tell you.

Those are my 26 reasons for being interested in self-defense. All of these stories are true, and all happened to me, to members of my family, to my neighbors or to my friends. *And we live in a low-crime neighborhood!* My interest in self-defense is based on an appreciation of the violence found in real life. If you disagree and find me to be a paranoid person, you'd be well advised to put this book down and read no farther. **Black Medicine** is a deadly art which does not spare the feelings of the squeamish.

N. Mashiro
June, 1979

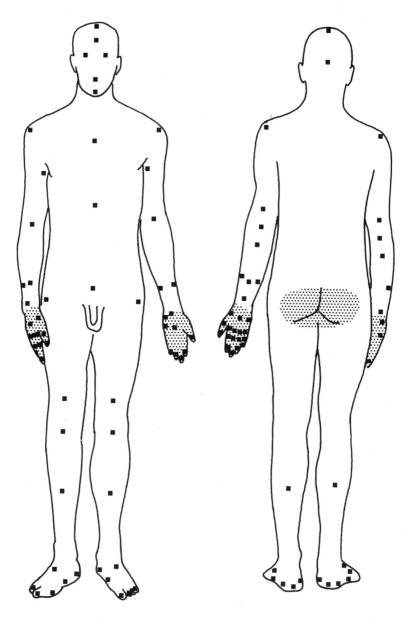

Fig. 1: There are natural weapons situated throughout the body. Although they are concentrated in the hands, it is literally true that if you can reach your opponent with any part of your body you can hurt him! (Compare this figure with the corresponding diagram of vulnerable areas of the body in *Black Medicine, The Dark Art of Death.*)

THE STRIKING POINTS

The striking points are the 112 parts of the body which martial artists use as weapons. Most of the striking points are concentrated in the hands and arms, but a substantial number are distributed throughout the body. Since you have natural weapons in every part of your body, *if you can reach your opponent with any part of your body you can hurt him*!

Figure 1 is a general overview of the parts of the body which may be used as weapons. These parts are discussed in detail on subsequent pages. The purpose of Figure 1 is simply to illustrate the point that there are natural weapons all over the body.

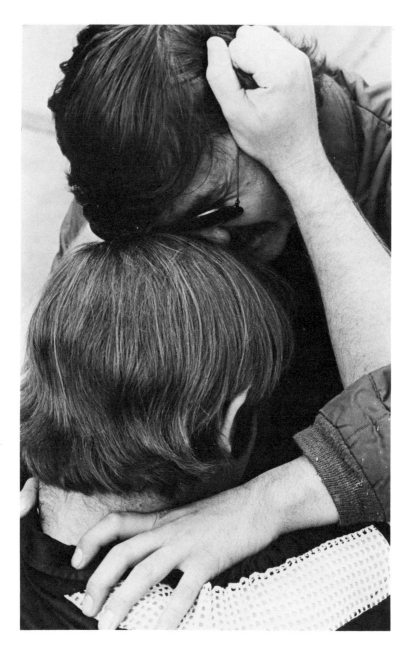

Fig. 2: The top of the head can be used as an anvil against which you may mash an opponent's face.

STRIKING POINTS
OF THE HEAD

Top of Head: The very top of the cranial vault, centered on the anterior two inches of the sagittal suture. This is the area where you would balance a book on top of your head. This area is actually not a very good natural weapon because butting the opponent with your head places a severe strain on your neck, both in terms of lateral twisting and simple compression of the vertebrae. Butting is commonly seen in soccer and in football, but karateists see it most often in the movies. Still, such an attack can be effective if the opponent is taken by surprise in the lower adbomen or groin. If you were bound to a chair being interrogated you might be able to throw yourself (and the chair) forward and deliver this blow. (See Figure 2.)

Forehead: The striking point is the center of the frontal bone, about two inches above the eyebrows. The frontal bone is a dome-like shield in the front of the skull which can receive tremendous impacts without damage. One frequently sees karateists showing off by breaking huge blocks of ice or stacks of bricks by striking them with the forehead. In combat the forehead is most useful for striking the opponent's nose, mouth, jaw or collarbone when your hands are pinned or bound.

Back of Head: The occipital bone in the vicinity of the lambdoid suture. This is not as good a striking point as the forehead because too strong an impact here can fracture the lambdoid suture and depress the occipital bone into the brain. The back of the head is almost always used to attack the nose and face of an assailant who has pinned your arms from behind. This situation is frequently encountered when one person holds you while another beats you from the front. Ramming your head backward into the opponent's nose and mouth may cause him enough pain to break his grip on your arms and body.

11

Chin: The bony tip of the mandible. Although the jaw is extremely strong it is not normally used for striking a blow because it connects directly with the balancing organs in the ear. Any jarring of the jaw, therefore, disrupts balance. The chin can be used for gouging, however. In a desperate one-on-one fight when your arms and legs are otherwise occupied (as in the deadlocked wrestling or judo match) the chin can be used to gouge at nerve centers within reach of the head. There are many such centers in the neck and shoulders, for instance, and chin pressure against the inguinal region can effect an immediate release from a scissors hold (see **Black Medicine, Vol. I** for nerve pressure points).

Teeth: Usually the upper and lower incisors, but can include molars under rare circumstances. The human jaw and teeth can deliver shearing and crushing forces in excess of 400 pounds per square inch. The incisors exert the least pressure and are best adapted to cutting or tearing, while the molars in the back of the jaw produce the strongest crushing forces. It is obvious that an opponent who puts his hand over your mouth (to silence you) is in danger of a bitten finger, and if you can work one of his fingers into the back of your mouth you can crush it between the rear molars. In a grappling or wrestling contest the teeth can be brought to bear on the opponent's ears, nose, lips, carotid sinus, thyroid cartilage and most nerve pressure points. Some karate schools teach a technique for attacking the throat which consists of butting the opponent in the face with your forehead, and as his head jerks back away from the blow you twist to the side and bite his Adam's apple. Tasty! (See Figure 3.)

Mind, Eyes and Voice: Your mind, eyes and voice are among your most powerful weapons, through which you can directly attack the opponent's mind without recourse to such crude methods as striking him physically. Training to use these mental weapons is the essence of true, traditional karate, and is one of the sad losses associated with the evolution of this art into a popular "sport." A master of this technique can paralyze you with the look in his eyes, or fill your mind with terror at the sound of his voice. This sounds improbable to the western mind, but the author has personally met many karateists who could knock a person off balance with a hostile facial expression alone.

My own mastery of the technique is limited, but I have employed it successfully in real life. On one occasion I confronted the leader of a small group of men who were intent on separating me from property which I was storing for a friend. My friend's belongings were not mine to give, and I said so. The leader of the gang was rather larger than I, and tried to get his way by growling dark threats and crowding me as the others watched and laughed. When we were about a foot apart he saw the look in my eyes and suddenly stopped. His face turned pale and he began to back away again. Stammering something

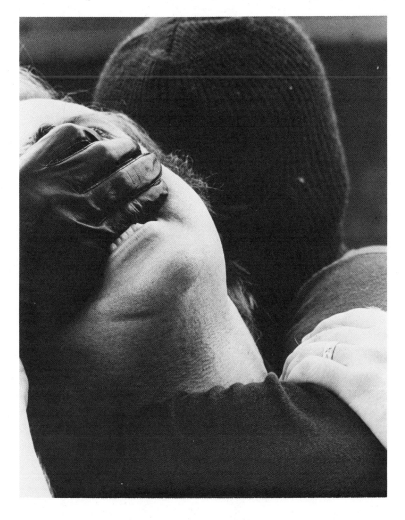

Fig. 3: **A person who clamps his hand over your mouth is asking for trouble. Use your teeth to make an impression on him.**

13

about coming back later, he led his gang away. He never bothered me again, but I heard later that he was in prison for murdering a defenseless storekeeper during a robbery. The look in my eyes had stopped him. It is a very valuable weapon.

Everyone has seen martial artists who shout insanely as they attack. This is a more obvious version fo the same psychological intimidation. But a loud shout isn't enough. The shout must possess emotional content in order to be effective. You may imagine this in terms of a shout of rage, or a shout of hatred, but a trained karateist can produce the same psychological effect when his mind is actually calm and rational. This karate shout, or *kiai*, can force a whole room full of people to step back involuntarily if they are not expecting it. I've seen it happen. The effect of this shout when directed against a single opponent at close range can be devastating.

STRIKING POINTS
OF THE ARMS & HANDS

Shoulder: The striking point is the acromial end of the scapular spine where it forms the bony "point" of the shoulder. The shoulder padding worn by football players is adequate testimony of the damage which this point can do when forcefully driven into an opponent's body. The point of the shoulder is usually employed against an opponent's solar plexus, floating ribs, bladder or genitals in a motion resembling a diving tackle. In judo contests one occasionally sees the shoulder being used to sneak in an illegal blow during an apparent throwing attempt. If the judges are not very alert such fouling can easily win many matches.

Armpit: Some high school wrestling teams boast that they win by "armpit power," by which they mean that the suffocate their opponents by not bathing. Here the reference is to the axillary area when it is used to clamp an opponent's arm or neck tightly against the side of the body. There are several elbow locks and throws which involve the armpit as a clamp or fulcrum.

Point of Elbow: The striking point is the olecranon, the sharp protuberance of the ulna where it forms the hard tip of the bent elbow. With the arm fully bent, the point of the elbow can be used to strike a very powerful blow either straight back into the opponent's ribs, or straight down into a bowing opponent's head and back. (Envision someone who is trying to tackle you around the waist. The elbow blow comes straight down into the back of his neck.) The point of the elbow is also used to strike straight out to the side, but this technique is rarely seen. It requires a lot of training to be powerful enough for serious applications. (See Figure 4.)

Front of Elbow: This term refers to the medial surface of the ulna within 3 inches of the point of the elbow. This is the hard,

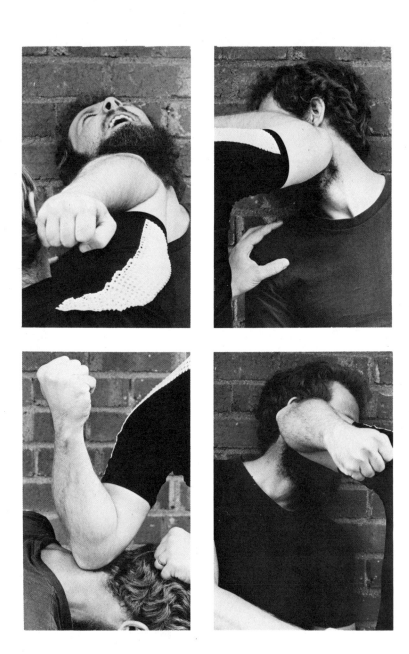

Fig. 4: The front of the elbow can kill when driven up under the opponent's chin *(top left).* It can also be used laterally, breaking the opponent's jaw *(top right).* The elbow point employed in a downward blow to the cervical vertebrae can easily break your opponent's neck *(below left).* The back of the elbow in a lateral strike to the opponent's head *(below right).*

bony surface of the forearm just beneath the joint. This surface is used to strike an "elbow blow" directly forward into the opponent's solar plexus, directly up under his chin, or horizontally into the side of his face. (Specifically, the attacker's right elbow moves horizontally from the attacker's right to left, hitting the left side of the defender's face.) These are extremely powerful infighting blows which do not require any special training to be effective. The rising blow under the chin is especially noteworthy, and can break the opponent's jaw or even his neck.

Back of Elbow: The posterior, distal end of the humerus, within 3 inches of the trochlea. This is the back of the upper arm just above the elbow. The back of the elbow is used to strike horizontally at the head or ribs of an attacker who has embraced you from behind, leaving your arms free. You twist sideways and swing the back of the elbow horizontally into the opponent's face. It can also be used as a backhand elbow blow against an opponent who is in front of you. A typical attack consists of using the *front* of the elbow to hit the left side of the opponent's face, then recoiling back using the *back* of the elbow to strike his face a second time.

Bend of Elbow: The anterior surface of the arm within four inches of the cubital fossa. The bend of the elbow cannot be used to strike an opponent, strictly speaking, but as a choking or strangulating device it is unsurpassed. The purest form involves wrapping your arm around the opponent's neck from behind and catching his Adam's apple directly in the fold of the arm. In this position the biceps in the upper arm and the many muscles of the forearm bear directly against the carotid arteries in the opponent's neck. A tight application of the hold cuts off the blood flow to the brain and the victim passes out almost immediately. The fold of the elbow is also used very often as a headlock, in which the opponent's head is held tightly at the side of your body while you strike him or otherwise deal with him.

Inside Edge of Forearm: The medial side of the forearm, especially the distal four inches of the ulna. This is the edge of the forearm on the same side as the little finger. A very common karate block (*tettsui-uke*) consists of deflecting an opponent's punch by striking his fist or arm with the inside edge of your forearm. The block consists of holding the forearm vertically (fist up, elbow down) and sweeping it across in front of the face or body to deflect the incoming punch.

Outside Edge of Forearm: The thumb edge of the forearm, especially the distal four inches of the radius. This surface is used for blocking similarly to the inside of the forearm, but the block begins with the fist in front of the opposite shoulder and sweeps back across the body.

Back of Forearm: The posterior surface of the forearm. This is the side of the wrist/forearm continuous with the back of the hand (where most people wear a watch). This surface is not commonly used in karate, the sides of the forearms being preferred for most purposes. The back of the forearm is most often used to break a front choke in which the opponent is squeezing your neck with both hands while standing in front of you. The release consists of clasping your hands together and driving the wedge formed by your forearms up between the opponent's arms. In this case it is the back of your forearms which strike the opponent's arms and break the hold.

Fingernails: We are all familiar with the fact that fingernails can be used for scratching, an ineffective technique at best. They can also be used for *clawing,* however, which is more practical. In this context the nails can be used to achieve deep penetration into the eyes, throat and especially the nerve pressure points on the back of the hand (see **Black Medicine, Vol. I**). Some dedicated karate and kung-fu artists allow their nails to grow 1/4 to 1/2 inch long, and strengthen them with nail hardener. Naturally they also sandpaper the tips to a sharp edge. The wound produced by four of these nails slashed across a person's throat (like saw teeth) is difficult to believe even when seen.

Tip of Thumb: The tip of the distal phalanx of the thumb, together with the sharp edge of the nail. The tip of the thumb is used for gouging, usually at the opponent's eyes but frequently involving the throat and other nerve pressure points. The trapezius muscle is especially vulnerable to a thumb gouge (see **Black Medicine, Vol. I** and Figure 5).

Foreknuckle of Thumb: The distal end of the proximal phalanx of the thumb. The foreknuckle of the thumb (immediately behind the thumbnail) can be used for jabbing into soft tissues. With the hand open, align the thumb in its natural position along the side of the hand. Now bend just the tip of the thumb in toward the palm, leaving the foreknuckle exposed. In this position you can use this striking point to attack the side of the opponent's throat. Jab your hand (palm down) along the side of the opponent's neck. Let your index finger slide along the

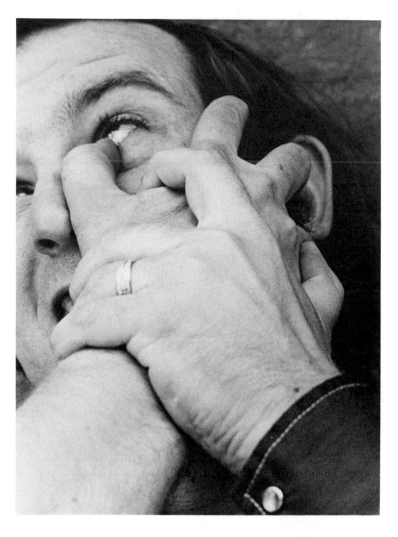

Fig. 5: The tip of the thumb and the thumbnail are excellent for gouging at an eyeball.

angle between his throat and jaw. This will guide the thumb knuckle directly into the carotid sinus. This is one of the most certain ways of hitting this small but very valuable nerve center.

Back of Thumb: Counting back from the thumb nail, the first joint is the foreknuckle, the second is the knuckle, and the "back of the thumb" is the bony area between the knuckle and the wrist. (The dorsal side of the first metacarpal bone.) When the hand is in the standard open attack position with the thumb pulled down into a tight knot next to the palm, the back of the thumb forms a hard bony ridge protruding at a 45 degree angle from the line of the forearm. This surface is usually employed in blocking, especially since the angle between the thumb and forearm can lock on to an opponent's wrist (behind his fist) and not only deflect his punch but pull him off balance.

Thumb and Forefinger: Which of us does not know how to pinch with thumb and forefinger? This pinch can be very painful when applied in the lip or nose region, and can crush a testicle like a soft-boiled egg. When the pinch catches the thyroid cartilage in its grip it can actually be fatal. (See Figure 6.)

Sides of Thumb and Forefinger: When the thumb is held out away from the open hand the "V" between it and the forefinger becomes a useful weapon for attacking the carotid sinuses in the throat. (See Figure 7.) The web of the thumb is rammed against the thyroid cartilage, and the sides of the thumb and forefinger strike against the sides of the neck in exactly the right location to shock the carotid baroreceptors and produce unconsciousness. (See **Black Medicine, Vol. I** for a discussion of the vulnerability of the carotid nerve centers.)

Tip of Forefinger: The tip of the distal phalanx of the first finger. Many karate schools teach a technique called *ippon-nukite*, the one-finger spearhand attack. In this attack the forefinger is held rigidly extended with the other three fingers partially bent beneath it, giving the forefinger strong support. This weapon is used to stab into the opponent's eye, throat or solar plexus. The attack is effective in proportion to the attacker's training. Anybody can poke his finger in someone's eye with a reasonable chance of success, but the attack to the solar plexus requires conditioning and training. (See Figure 8.)

Tips of Forefinger and Middle Finger: The tips of the distal phalanges of the first and second fingers. The fingers are usually spread about two inches apart and are used for stabbing into the opponent's eyes. This is the famous "Three Stooges" eye attack, but it is not formed in the common V-for-

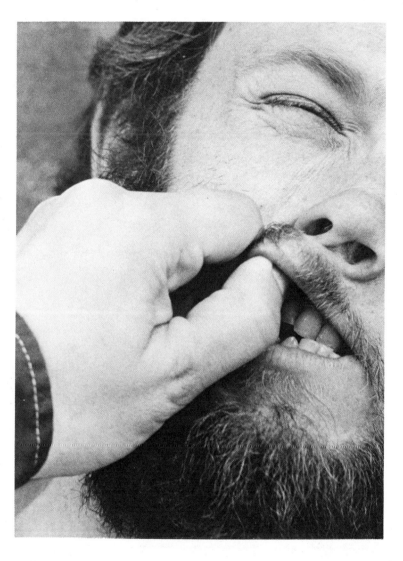

Fig. 6: The pinch of the thumb and forefinger is best applied to the lip, nose, or the Adam's apple.

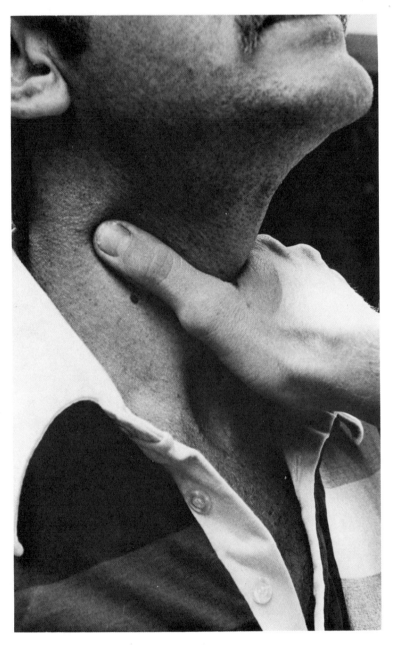

Fig. 7: The 'V' between the thumb and the edge of the palm can be rammed up into a person's throat, doing damage to the thyroid cartilage and both carotid nerve centers. The result is unconsciousness or even death, but with little risk of injury to the hand.

victory finger position. The forefinger and middle finger are fully extended, but the ring and little fingers are only half bent and serve to support the middle finger. Sometimes the thumb is laid along side of the forefinger to give it additional support, too. A karateist trained in finger spearing techniques can stab through the eye sockets and into the brain with this technique. (See Figure 8.)

Tips of Forefinger, Middle and Ring Fingers: The tips of the distal phalanges of the first, second and third fingers. This is the classic karate "spear hand" attack, which consists of holding the fingers, hand and wrist as straight and stiff as a board while ramming the ends of the fingers into the opponent's throat, solar plexus or even his ribs. There are several minor variations in the technique. In most cases the fingers are held tightly together with the middle finger slightly bent to make the three fingers about the same length. In another method the finger tips form a triangle, with the middle finger resting on top of the appressed fore and ring fingers. In yet another method the fingers are spread with about an inch of space between each finger tip. (This arrangement is for attacking the trachea or the eyes when you want to be sure you don't miss.) Another version involves bending the fingers into a sharp right angle with the hand. The wrist is also bent back slightly, which makes the position of the hand resemble a "Z" in shape. In the days of old when karateists trained for years to toughen their hands, it was said that a true practitioner of the art could stab through a man's body wall with this technique. There are only a few people today who can accomplish this feat, but they are sincerely respected. (See Figure 8.)

Tips of Fore, Middle, Ring and Little Fingers: Hold your hand open, with the fingers extended straight but with a one inch gap between the middle and ring fingers. In some karate schools this position is called an "extractor" hand, because it can be thrust palm-up into the opponent's groin. The two groups of fingers pass on either side of his penis and direct all their force into the testicles.

Little Finger: In many Army manuals you will find the comment that the little finger is a lethal weapon. This is preposterous. The comment usually alludes to the knife-hand chop (discussed below) which uses the little-finger *edge of the palm*, which is not the same thing as the little finger at all. As we all know, however, the little finger is precisely the right size to insert into a nostril, and the effect on an opponent's state of

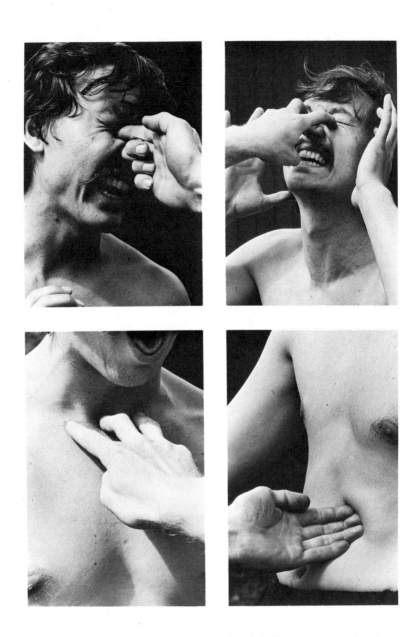

Fig. 8: The one-finger attack to the eye *(top left)*. Two fingers used to attack the eyes *(top right)*. Three fingers in a stab to the throat. At least one finger will crush the trachea even if the attack is partially deflected *(below left)*. The full spear-hand attack to the floating ribs. Some experts drive their fingers in under the ribs, then grasp the lower ribs and pull *(below right)*.

mind when you insert *your* finger into *his* nostril is devastating. The finger-in-the-nose technique is one of the simplest and most effective releases from an unwanted embrace.

Foreknuckle of Forefinger: The distal end of the proximal phalanx first finger. The "foreknuckles" are those which one uses to knock on a door. When the hand is clenched into a fist the forefinger can be unfolded slightly so that the foreknuckle forms a point. This point is used to gouge or stab sharply at nerve centers and other small vital points, such as the temple, philtrum, solar plexus and any of several nerve centers in the throat (see **Black Medicine, Vol. I**).

Foreknuckle of Middle Finger: The distal end of the proximal phalanx of the second finger. The foreknuckle of the middle finger can be allowed to protrude from a clenched fist similarly to that of the forefinger, discussed above. It is employed identically to the foreknuckle of the forefinger except that the middle finger is better supported and can confidently be used to strike a little harder than in the previous case.

Foreknuckles of Fore, Middle, Ring and Little Fingers: The distal ends of the proximal phalanges of all the fingers. Imagine jabbing at the opponent's throat with your fingertips. Now fold your fingers as if starting to make a fist and jab with the foreknuckles instead (the knuckles you use for knocking on a door). These knuckles form a hard, penetrating weapon which is especially useful in slipping a punch in under the chin to the soft tissues of the throat. This technique is also used against the philtrum, temple, solar plexus and the subaxillary nerve bundle in the armpit. (See **Black Medicine, Vol. I** for discussion of these nerve centers.)

Knuckles: The distal ends of the second and third, or the second through fifth metacarpal bones. (The first metacarpal bone is in the thumb, the second is at the base of the forefinger, etc.) These are the knuckles we instinctively use when striking with a clenched fist. There are two ways to form the first, depending on whether you prefer the boxing approach or the karate approach. In boxing the fist is formed with all four knuckles aligned to hit the target at the same time. The karate version concentrates force into the knuckles of the fore and middle fingers by folding the ring and little fingers farther back into the fist. The fist is used to punch at the opponent's face, throat, abdomen, groin, kidneys and other soft parts of the body. Trained karateists can deliver extremely powerful punches even against hard parts of the body, fracturing the skull, sternum and ribs with equal facility. Do not make the common mistake of punching the opponent in the jaw, however, unless you really know what you are doing. It is much too easy to break bones in your fist when you strike such a strong, angular bone as the mandible.

Back of Fist: A very common karate blow involves a backhand strike using the knuckle fore and middle finger. This attack is usually directed at the temple of the face in a very fast snapping motion.

Bottom of Fist: The medial side of the fifth metacarpal, together with fleshy tissues appertaining. The little-finger side of a clenched fist can be used like a hammer to deliver extremely powerful blows, especially against the opponent's head, collarbone, forearms, legs and groin. Japanese karate teachers call this the *tettsui*, or iron hammer. When used to block an incoming punch, the iron hammer blow can literally break the other man's arm.

Palm of Hand: When the hand is open the flat palm is the natural weapon preferred for such non-injurious attacks as slapping and spanking. It produces less innocuous results, however, when directed at the nose, groin, or when clapped over the outer opening of the ear canal.

Folded Palm: Touch your little finger to your thumb, and notice the fold which appears in the palm from the heel of the hand up to the base of the forefinger. This is the basis for one of the "sticky hands" techniques in which the opponent's punch is not only blocked, but actually *caught and held* in mid-strike. The block is accomplished with the palm loosely folded. As the opponent's left fist comes in toward your head, you block with your right hand, allowing his forearm to enter the semi-circle of your palm and fingers. The narrow "V" of the folded palm slides freely down his forearm, but locks tight when it encounters his wrist. This capture is usually seen in conjunction with a judo throw or footsweep. (See Figure 9.)

Heel of Palm: When the wrist is bent back the heel of the hand becomes a most formidable impact weapon. The palm heel can be used for punching attacks to the jaw, nose, solar plexus, ribs and groin. The advantage of using the palm heel is that it is less subject to injury than the knuckles, and there is no danger of spraining the wrist. Also, a person must be properly trained to punch correctly with his fists, but palm heel attacks can be learned almost instantly.

Back of Hand: When the hand is open, the bony back of the hand can be used for especially painful slapping, and in karate it is also used for deflecting incoming punches.

Edge of Hand: The "chop," one of the most famous karate or judo blows, is delivered with the little-finger edge of the palm. The hand is held open with the thumb folded down tightly, almost as if you were trying to touch the thumb tip to the center of the palm. (Many military manuals show this position incorrectly with the thumb extended away from the hand.) The striking surface is the medial side of the fifth metacarpal, and

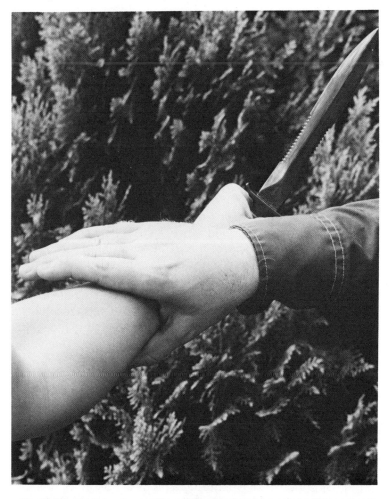

Fig. 9: **The folded palm position of the hand looks weak and loose, but in practice it is an excellent way to ensnare the opponent's arm in mid-strike. The V-shaped cavity formed by the hand slips easily along the opponent's forearm, but locks tightly when it reaches his wrist.**

27

the associated fleshy tissue. The "knife-hand" attack usually does not involve the little finger or the first inch of palm at the little finger's base, but is focused on the fleshier two-thirds of the palm's edge. This attack is especially favored among martial artists because it concentrates the force of the blow into an area of only two or three square inches. The "chop" is most effective against the temple, nose, throat, neck, collarbone, several points on the forearm, and the inside of the thigh.

Ridge Hand: This is an "edge of the hand" technique which uses the second metacarpal bone instead of the fifth. With the hand held open and the thumb tucked down deeply into the palm, the edge of the hand at the base of the index finger can be used to strike at the temple, side of neck, floating ribs and groin. This technique is frequently seen in professional "karate" tournaments where it is delivered with a flailing motion. The attacker swings his shoulder past the target, allowing his arm to follow like a whip. Although striking with the inside edge of the hand would seem to be a very weak and limited technique, once mastered it is very powerful and can be employed frequently in karate matches.

Lower Edge of Hand: A modified form of the "knife hand" attack consists of bending the whole hand slightly back at the wrist and then slightly down (in the direction of the little finger). This special blow is designed to break the collarbone, and uses only the edge of the *heel* of the hand for striking.

Back of Wrist: The distal ends of the radius and ulna on their posterior (dorsal) surface. Bend your hand and wrist as if trying to touch your fingertips to the inside of your wrist. In this position the back of the wrist presents a hard surface which is used for several blocks and strikes, especially to the face. This striking point converts a simple backhand slap into a punishing blow.

Whole Hand: While discussing the many small parts of the hand which can be used as weapons, it is important to remember that the functions of the *whole* hand can be weapon-like, too. The simple act of grasping is used very frequently in combat, to hold and pull an opponent's wrist, clothing or hair. Some of the more heavily built karateists can break a person's forearm by grasping it around the wrist and squeezing! Grasping the opponent's sleeve during a block is very common, and controlling his head by grasping his ears or hair is an extremely effective technique. All depend on the use of the whole hand in its role as a grasping instrument.

STRIKING POINTS
OF THE TORSO

Chest: The chest is not normally used as a striking surface, but in exceptional circumstances it can be quite effective. One thinks of a bully using his chest to push his victim around, but the chest can also be used as an anvil into which you can pull the opponent's face. The sternum seems very hard and unforgiving when your nose hits it at high speed. Also, the size of a man's chest is an effective psychological dominance asset. Large men who "puff up" their chests when annoyed are rarely attacked.

Abdomen: In karate, the abdomen is considered to be the center of all power. This concept is usually taught as a semi-mystical belief, but there is a sound anatomical basis for it as well. All attacks delivered with the arms and hands become much more powerful when firmly driven from a solid base. If the abdomen is not tense and inflexible at the moment of impact, much of the power of the attack is absorbed in rotating the upper trunk relative to the feet and hips (a recoil motion). The abdomen is not necessarily a *source* of physical power, but unless it is held rigid at the moment of impact it does act as a *sink*, draining power away from the blow. Mastery of the ability to "focus" an attack for maximum power involves considerable abdominal coordination, and is the single most valuable technique an unarmed fighter can possess.

Hips: Taken here to mean the lateral projections of the femurs, not the iliac crest. The extreme upper part of the side of the thigh, opposite the hip joint. The hip is a striking point in judo and jui-jitsu. It is used like a battering ram during the initial motion of many throws to break the opponent's balance and posture. The force of this blow can be appreciated by the fact that it is possible to break several boards with this hip impact alone. The effect when the blow catches the opponent squarely in the groin is very dramatic. Most people will dive right into the throw rather than try to resist the full power of this attack.

There is another meaning of "using the hips" which is more typical of karate. This meaning implies locking the hips rigidly at the moment of impact of a hand or foot blow. The reasons are similar to those discussed for locking the abdomen at the same time (see above).

Buttocks: The buttocks are among the strongest and most heavily padded parts of the body. This is the reason they are preferred for the ritualized striking of naughty children, since there is very little possibility of injury other than bruising. The buttocks, however, can actually be employed as a lethal weapon under the right circumstances. When held around the waist from behind, a person can bend down, grasp the attacker's ankle, jerk it up and spill him on his back. At that point if you violently drop your whole weight on his chest (buttocks first) you can squash him like a bug. A crushed rib cage is an extremely serious injury. Who would have thought that the lowly bottom could be so deadly?

Groin: One of the more colorful episodes of my karate training occurred when an instructor became confused one day and finished an explanation with this remarkable statement: "Then you finish him off by slamming your groin into his knee!" Poor advice. In judo, however, the pubis bone (the hard bone you can feel just above the genitals) is commonly used as a fulcrum for various elbow locks. If you have thrown your opponent on his back you can lock his elbow by holding the back of his wrist next to your navel and levering back against his elbow. The back of the elbow is thrust forward by the pubis bone, locking the arm and producing considerable pain (for him, not you!).

STRIKING POINTS
OF THE LEG & FOOT

Front of Thigh: The front of the thigh within eight inches of the knee can be used for a groin attack during very close in-fighting. The blow resembles that of a knee-strike into the opponent's groin, but is used when you are too close to effectively use your knee.

Knee: The knee is almost as versatile as the elbow when it comes to striking powerful blows in a variety of directions. The most obvious attack is the classic knee in the groin, which is usually a straight-in type of blow. The knee can also be used for a rising blow, as when you grasp the opponent's hair with your hands and pull his head down into your rising knee. Karateists quickly learn to deliver roundhouse knee attacks, in which the knee is cocked out to the side of the body and swept in a horizontal arc into the side of the opponent's body. In this case the targets selected are usually the abdomen or rib cage. In the case of an opponent who has been thrown to the ground, dropping on his body with one or both knees can be extremely damaging. Lastly, the knee is frequently used to ward off or deflect incoming kicks. Note that in this application the knee is fully flexed and held high in front of the groin as a shield. (See Figure 10.)

Shin: The front of the lower leg is sometimes used for kicks to the groin, rib cage, or side when the distance to the target is too great for a knee attack but too short for a proper kick. The attack against the genitals is especially effective, since the shin is very hard and the target offers no possibility of injury to the leg.

Calf: The back of the lower leg is used in some of the simpler judo throws in which you throw the opponent by stepping to his side and sweeping his legs out from under him from behind using the back of your leg. The back of the thigh is also used in this way.

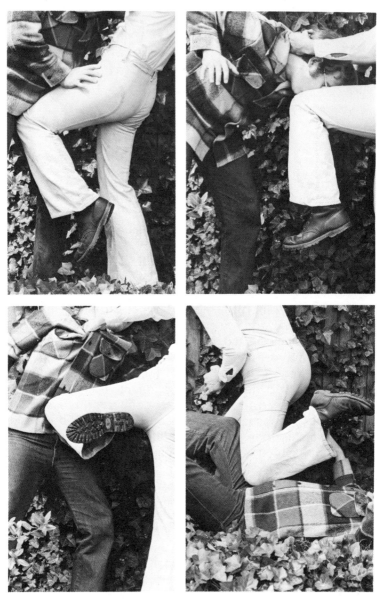

Fig. 10: The classic knee attack to the groin. Notice the ineffective block *(top left)*. When the opponent folds after the groin attack, a follow-up attack to the face is easy to apply *(top right)*. The knee can also be used in a roundhouse manner. Here the opponent is trapped between the incoming knee, and fence *(below left)*. Finally, the knee can be used to strike a blow directly downward. Drop on the opponent, driving your knee deep into his chest or abdomen *(below right)*.

Top of Foot: The tarsus and metatarsal bones on the dorsal surface of the foot. With the foot fully extended (as if standing on your toes) the bony upper surface between the ankle and the toes can be used to attack the groin, floating ribs, head and face. This is especially easy in terms of the groin, because like the thigh and shin the top of the foot does not require exact placement in order to damage the genitals. Attacks to the ribs and head usually involve roundhouse kicks. These kicks begin with the foot and leg cocked horizontally to the side, from which the foot is whipped in a horizontal or ascending arc to the target. More rarely a flying kick is used. This is similar to the roundhouse kick in general, and the biggest difference being that you lightly spring four or five feet up into the air first.

Ball of Foot: With the ankle and toes fully *extended* (as if trying to touch your toes to the front of your shin) the ball of the foot becomes properly positioned for use as a natural weapon. Actually the position of the ankle varies from one kick to another, but the toes are always bent up as far as possible to avoid breaking them between the ball of the foot and the target. Kicks using the ball of the foot can strike upward into the kneecap, groin, solar plexus, armpit, throat or chin. If the knee is raised high during the kick the attack may come almost straight in, striking the abdomen or groin. When used with a roundhouse kick the ball of the foot can inflict very severe damage to the skull and rib cage. This is one of the most powerful and most frequently used of all karate weapons.

Toes: The toes are not usually involved in kicks because they are too easily sprained, dislocated and broken. They can be used in a kick to the genitals where reaching the target is more important than delivering a really powerful blow. A kick which hooks around the opponent's thigh and jars the testicles *from behind* is an example of this kind of attack. Of course the "toe" of a shoe is a perfectly respectable striking device. (See Figure 11.)

Bottom of Foot: The entire ventral surface of the foot, normally in contact with the ground while standing. The bottom of the foot is used in some simple backward kicks (think of a donkey) and in stamping attacks against the opponent's toes. When you are squared off against another karateist you can frequently nullify his tactics by stepping on his leading foot and pinning it to the ground. When he involuntarily glances down at his foot you can exploit his inattention with a hand attack to the head.

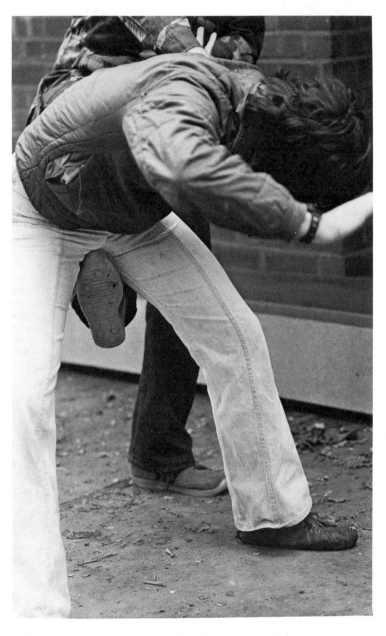

Fig. 11: The toes are rarely used as striking points because of their fragility. Against the genitals, however, the toes perform very effectively.

Sole of Foot: By "sole" is meant that part of the bottom of the foot which corresponds anatomically to the palm of the hand. In a *crescent kick* you swing your foot in a high rising arc which passes up one side of the opponent's body, across his face, and back down to the ground on the other side. The blow is like slapping the face with the sole of your foot. Crescent kicks are also used against the opponent's hands (to deflect weapons) and against his chest. The sole of the foot is commonly used in footsweep attacks, too, in which you "slap" the opponent's feet out from under him using the sole of your foot.

Outer Edge of Foot: Stand with your foot flat on the floor. Turn your ankle sideways to roll the foot over onto its outer edge. This sharp edge of the foot is used in karate thrust kicks against the opponent's instep, shin, knee, thigh, groin, abdomen, ribs, throat and skull (see **Black Medicine Vol I.** for details). The narrowness of this part of the foot concentrates the power of the attack into such a small space that all the force can be concentrated on *one* rib, for instance. With the entire mass of the powerful leg muscles behind it, such a kick produces astonishing penetration and internal damage.

Upper Edge of Foot: The "upper" edge of the foot is a narrow band of tissue roughly overlying the fifth metatarsal bone. It is on *top*, running along the outer edge from the base of the little toe to the heel. When the edge of the foot is used in rising kicks against the chin, groin, armpit, elbows and hands the striking area is not quite the same as in the case of a thrust kick. (For the true karateist, the kick envisioned here is the side snap kick, or *yoko geri keage*).

Inner Edge of Foot: The inner side of the foot, running from the big toe back to the ankle, is not as effective in kicks as the outer edge, but it's natural curvature helps the foot cling to the opponent's shin during an attack on the lower leg and foot. You swing your foot in to attack his shin, contacting with the inner edge of your foot and bruising the nerves in his shin. Then you drive your foot downward along the length of the shin bone until the bottom of your foot crushes his instep. A very effective attack, especially when wearing shoes.

Bottom of Heel: Persons who are especially limber can deliver a kick in which the blow is delivered with the bottom of the heel alone. This is accomplished by driving the foot straight in to the opponent's chest with the ankle bent as far back toward the shin as possible. At the point of impact the opponent is struck by a solid column of bone extending from the pelvis to the heel. It feels very much like running at full speed into the end of a battering ram.

Side of Heel: In a *reverse* crescent kick the outer edge of the heel can be used to rake across the opponent's face. The kick involves bringing your right foot in a rising arc up the *right* side of the opponent's body, rapping him across the face with your heel, and then completing the circle to your original position.

Back of Heel: The back of the heel is used in the back snap kick against an opponent who is behind you. If the attacker has grabbed you from behind and pinned your arms, the back of the heel can be used with great effect against his shins, knee caps, and even his groin. There is one specialty kick in which you swing your leg as if to strike the opponent's side with the back of your knee. Instead, at the last second you bend your knee and strike him in the kidney *from behind* with the back of your heel! (See Figure 12.)

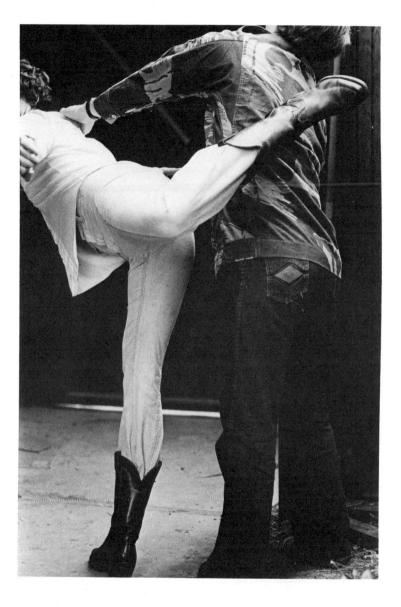

Fig. 12: The reverse roundhouse kick, delivered with the back of the heel, is one of the most unexpected karate attacks. It literally wraps around the opponent's body and strikes from behind.

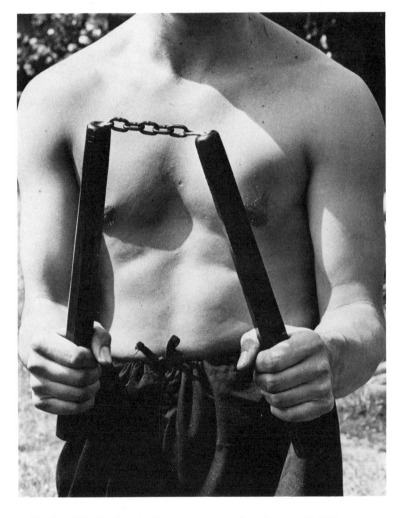

Fig. 13: **This classic oriental weapon was originally a rice flail. The conversion of a farming tool to a weapon illustrates the essence of makeshift weaponry.**

MAKESHIFT WEAPONS

The second half of the volume is devoted to a subject only one step removed from that of the body's natural weapons. This is the neglected topic of makeshift weapons. I call it a neglected topic because there has been very little effort made to refine our knowledge of makeshift weapons into a modern martial art. The most recent significant advances in this field are now over 100 years out of date.

The last period of creative development in the field of makeshift weaponry occurred in Okinawa in the 1800's. Conquering Japanese armies confiscated all "weapons" from the local population, including the household cooking knives! In response the Okinawans developed their knowledge of hand-to-hand combat and the use of makeshift weapons to a high art. Their new knowledge made their hands and feet very powerful, and their innocent-looking farming tools gradually began to serve double duty as surprisingly effective weapons. (This was a classic case of ploughshares forged into swords!) To this period of adversity we owe the development of modern karate and the development of several exotic oriental "weapons."

The best example of an oriental makeshift weapon is the *nunchaku.* This is a pair of wooden sticks, each about a foot long, which are joined at one end by a short length of chain or cord to form a formidable wooden whip or flail. (See Figure 13.) The nunchaku does terrible damage to an opponent, and has become popular in karate movies where the hero deftly pulls a nunchaku from his sleeve and uses it to defeat an army of attackers.

The nunchaku *is* a *makeshift* weapon. It is really an Okinawan rice-threshing flail, used to beat the grains of rice loose from the stalks on the threshing floor. The Japanese soldiers did not confiscate these threshing flails as weapons because they regarded them as harmless farming tools. The same situation applied to the *sai*, a short pitchfork used for handling bales of rice. It too became a very effective weapon, especially against sword-wielding soldiers.

Today, on the streets of many American cities, it is a felony to be found in possession of these oriental "weapons." The reason is simple. In modern America it is difficult to justify having a rice flail under one's coat for any purpose other than hitting people. The same can be said of carrying the pitchfork-like sai, the yawara stick (a former holy-water vessel carried by monks) or any of several other formerly useful makeshift weapons. These weapons were successful in their day because they were routinely at hand serving other purposes when trouble appeared. We would do well to emulate the ingenuity of the Okinawans and examine the perfectly legal objects we handle every day which might be developed into formidable weapons.

Makeshift weapons are common household items which can be used or converted into weapons on the spur of the moment. These objects are not normally thought of as weapons, and as such are usually available to a hostage or kidnap victim. Many of them can be placed near a door to repel an unwanted intruder, and others can be inconspicuously (and legally) carried about the person. The following list covers more than 180 such items, but should not be considered complete. The objects which can be used as makeshift weapons are limited only by the user's fighting skill and imagination. (See Figure 14.)

Alarm Clock: Any small appliance like an electric alarm clock can be swung by its power cord in imitation of a medieval mace-and-chain. Strike at the head and face, or let the cord wrap itself around the opponent's defending arm like a South American bola, then pull him off balance and follow through with a fist or foot attack.

Ashes: Wood ashes from a fireplace, or especially cigarette ashes from an ashtray. Throw a handful of white, powdery ashes into the opponent's face to blind and choke him.

Ashtray: Many of the large glass or ceramic ashtrays make heavy clubs. After throwing the ashes in his face, grasp the ashtray like a frisbee and hit him in the temple with the edge or corner.

Auto Antenna: An auto AM radio antenna can be broken off at the base, telescoped down to a compact size, and concealed in your waistband, trouser pocket or sock. In the compact form

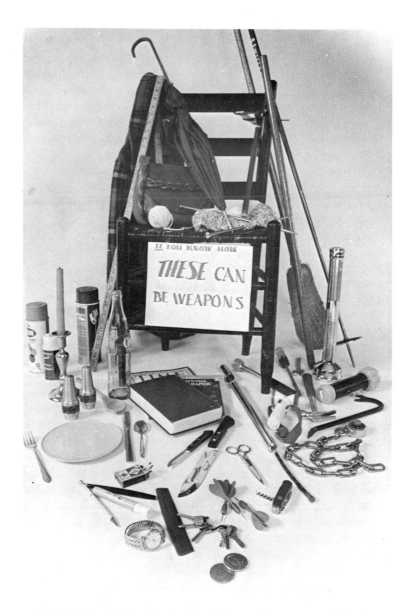

Fig. 14: In the right hands almost anything can be a weapon. This picture shows a selection of more than 180 makeshift weapons discussed in the following pages. *Everything* in the picture can be used to injure or kill when used correctly.

it can be used for stabbing at the eyes or gouging at nerve centers in the throat. Extended, the antenna can still be used in a surprise lunge at the eyes as well as being employed as a rapier-like whip. (Slash at the face.)

Axe: Remember Lizzie Borden? The edge of the axe is most effective if applied to the side of the skull, the back of the skull, the backbone just above the hips, and the area of the solar plexus. For the solar plexus attack try to catch the opponent as he is just entering the room. Stand beside the door and swing the axe horizontally like a baseball bat. That way the axe head will slip between the ribs on its way into the chest.

Axe Handle: A very convenient club, but best used for spear-like lunges with the end. The handle is actually a more versatile and handier weapon than the whole axe, so if you have time remove the axe head before using.

Bar of Soap: Sooner or later your captors will give you a bar of soap, if only to be relieved of the smell of you. Slip the soap inside your sock (or wrap it in a towel) and use it as a blackjack. Strike for the temple, for the mastoid process behind the ear, or for the collarbone. (See Figure 15.)

Baseball: Ever wonder why batters wear helmets, and umpires encase themselves in padding? A baseball is a very handy, very hard object which can do a lot of damage if propelled with enough force. Use it as a bludgeon or missile.

Baseball Bat: Used similarly to an axe handle, but the bat is heavier and slower. When fleeing from an attacker a very effective use of the bat is to sling it, spinning horizontally along the ground, into the attacker's legs. He will have a hard time avoiding a disabling shin injury. (Note: It is usually better not to throw away your weapon as a general policy.)

Basting Syringe: Who says that the terrorists won't come after you on Thanksgiving? A squirt of searing grease in the face from a basting syringe could be just the thing. The basting syringes with attached hypodermic needles can be used for injecting air or poison (drain cleaner and water) into the opponent's body. Air bubbles in an artery can be fatal.

Bath Towel: A bath towel can be used as a whip (visit any locker room and see for yourself), as a garrote, and as the handle for a soap blackjack. Tie the bar of soap in one corner of the towel and start swinging. Another possibility would be to fold the towel in half across its width and use it as a sling. Dump a can of hot pepper in the towel and sling the powder into your opponent's face.

42

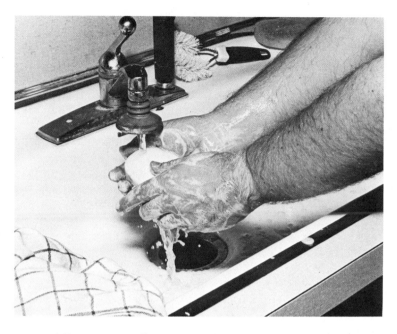

Fig. 15: If your captors allow you to wash your hands you will have access to all the materials you need for a soap-and-towel blackjack.

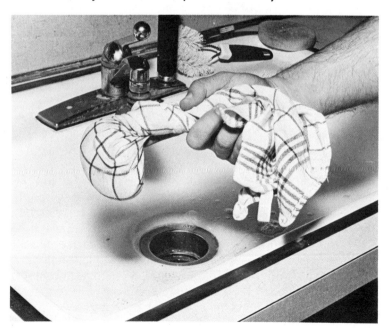

43

Baton: Is your daughter a cheerleader? Buy her a new baton after you rap the old one around the intruder's ears.

Beer Can: Shake it up a little and let it squirt into the captor's face as you pop the top. Then as he wipes his eyes you can dent the side of his skull with the bottom edge of the can. The cylindrical shape makes this edge surprisingly strong and hard even though the can itself is relatively flimsy. You can also crush the center of the can, bend it back and forth, and finally break it in two pieces. Grip one in each hand and smash the ragged edges into the bad guy's eyes.

Beer Mug: A heavy glass mug. When the local bully starts to push you around in the bar, you can propose a toast in his honor. Hold your mug aloft in salute, dump the beer on his head, and break his collarbone with the heavy glass base of the mug. The mug can also be used against the jaw and the bridge of the nose.

Belt: A belt is normally used as a whip or flail, frequently with the buckle swinging at the free end. It can also be used to strangle, or to tie up a prisoner. As a last resort, you can hang yourself with it.

Bicycle: If someone tries to abduct or rob you while you are cycling, you should realize that your bicycle itself is a powerful weapon. Just pick it up by the center of the handlebars and the back of the seat. Turn rapidly through one full turn to build up momentum and fling it, sprocket first, right in his face. A bicycle is an angular, hard, sharp, heavy object to see coming at you through midair. No one can be hit by one without suffering several injuries. (See Figure 16.)

Bicycle Chain: A bike chain is an old street fighter standby, because it is light, easy to conceal, blindingly fast in use, and produces vicious superficial wounds.

Bicycle Pump: Mount a tubular bicycle pump on the frame of the bike beneath the seat. Then if you see trouble ahead you can casually reach down and unfasten this excellent substitute for a police baton. And no one can accuse you of carrying it to use as a weapon! A bike has to have a pump, right? (See Figure 17.) If you are improvising and have some time to spare, pour some powdered cleanser or bleach into the pump. Then blow the chemicals into the opponent's face prior to hitting him.

Bleach: A cup of Clorox in the face does wonders to a person's ability to defend himself. When his hands fly up to his eyes you can kick him in a tender place.

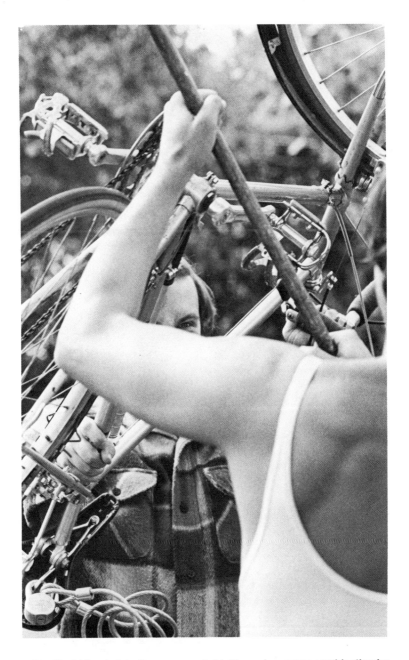

Fig. 16: A bicycle is both weapon and shield . . . a dangerous combination for any attacker to face. And while his eyes are on the upraised bike, you can easily kick him in the crotch.

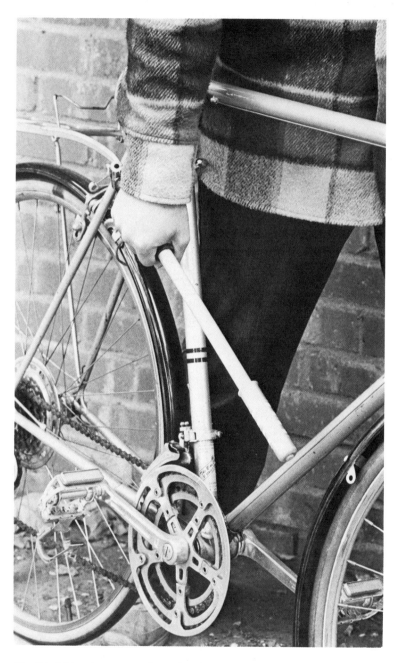

Fig. 17: A bicycle pump makes a handy nightstick when necessary.

46

Boiling Water: In the form of coffee, tea or soup. Slosh about a quart of it in the attacker's face or hands, then hit him over the head with the coffee pot (or soup pan).

Blender: When my editor first read over this manuscript he jokingly remarked that the only thing missing was the kitchen blender! "Stuff the kidnapper into the blender," he fantasized, "and set it for 'liquidate.'" After that remark I took a closer look at my blender, and found that the bottom of the blending chamber unscrews for cleaning the blades. The blade unit makes a nice, handy, "tiger paw" which would be very useful for slashing at an opponent's face.

Bones: Remember Samson and the jawbone of the ass? A soup bone can be a mighty club if necessary. If you have a whole skeleton to choose from (such as a horse skeleton) use the upper long bone of the foreleg, the *humerus*. Grasp the rounded shoulder end and strike with the knobby elbow end. The preferred weapon of our pre-human ancestors was an antelope humerus, but anyone you hit will probably fail to see the humer.

Books: Large, flat books make pretty effective shields against knife and fist attacks. Hold the book in both hands with the flat side facing the opponent. Alternately, a smaller book can be used to strike punishing blows at an attacker's arms, neck, collarbone and face. You can even gouge his eyes with the corners of the book. (See Figure 18.)

Boots: Especially pointed, high-heeled cowboy boots. The pointed toes give great penetration to toe kicks, and the heels do the same for kicks using the bottom of the foot. I was once in a karate demonstration where I played the bad guy who got stomped in the stomach by the cowboy in the white hat. His heels were a little longer than he thought. It made for a *very* realistic demonstration.

Bottle: A soft drink bottle is very strong, and can be used to stab or club an opponent. A thin-walled wine bottle is more useful when the base is shattered. Grasp it by the neck and stab or slash with the jagged broken end. Broken glass is the sharpest edge known to man.

Bowie Knife: A heavy bladed, hook-nose hunting knife. There is a whole school of knife fighting associated with these knives, characterized more by axe-like chopping than by slashing or stabbing. See Styers' **Cold Steel** for further information (available from Paladin Press).

Broom: The handle of a standard sweeping broom is good

for bayonet-like thrusts to the solar plexus and throat, and for deflecting incoming punches or knife attacks. The dusty straw end is very effective when jammed into a person's face. The stiff straws find their way into his mouth, nose and eyes all at once. To make that special impression, set fire to the straw first. (See Figure 19.)

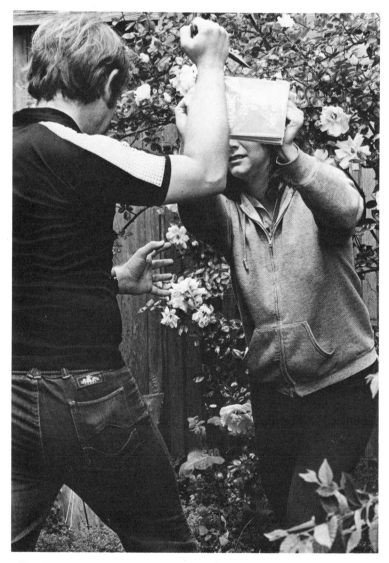

Fig. 18: A simple book can make a surprisingly effective shield against a knife attack.

Buckle: A star-shaped belt buckle about 3 inches in diameter is deadly when swung at the end of a belt. Buckles can also be used when detached from the belt as knuckle dusters, or clenched in the fist to provide a hard edge for gouging. The Bowen belt buckle knife is outstanding for this kind of thing. It is a sheath knife disguised as a belt buckle.

Cabinet Door: An open cabinet door represents several possibilities for a sudden attack on a captor or guard. If he opens a

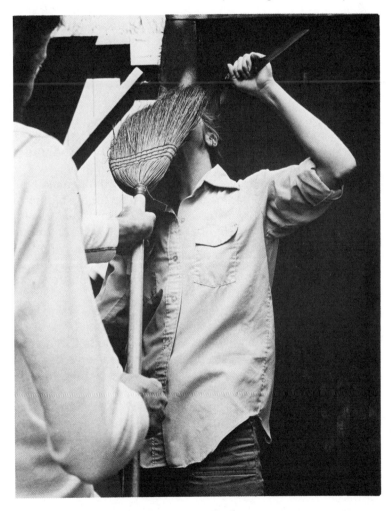

Fig. 19: **A broom is one of the most formidable household weapons. Not only does the handle possess all the qualities of a staff, but the dusty straws cause instant blindness when rammed into the eyes.**

cabinet and looks inside, slam the door *hard* against the back of his head. If he sticks his hand inside, slam the door on his fingers or wrist. Of course you can also slam a cabinet door *open* if you are looking inside the cabinet and the guard is standing next to you. If you are left alone in a room with wooden cabinets, wrench or kick a door off its hinges, split it by angling it against the wall and stomping on it, and use the resulting slats of wood as clubs.

Calculator: Many hand-held calculators are small enough to be grasped tightly in the fist and used to attack an intruder. Use the corner of the calculator in a vicious blow against the temple for maximum effect.

Camera: Nobody in his right mind would ruin a good camera by striking someone with it, right? So, be a little crazy and surprise the hell out of the bastard. Depending on the model, a camera can be opened up and used as a hinged flail or as a simple "blunt object." Detach the lens and use it to hammer on the other guy's head. If the camera has a built-in flash be sure to fire it in his eyes at close range before attacking.

Candle: A thick candle about ten inches long makes an effective short club. Imagine being locked up for the night in a basement cell with only a straw pallet and a smoky candle for company. Set the straw on fire, shout "Help! Fire!" and brain the guard with the hard, lower end of the candle when he gropes his way into the smoke-filled cell. Alternately, you can ram the lighted end into his face and let him concentrate on hot wax while you duck out the door.

Cane: The kind with a curved, hook-like handle. Aside from rapping the bad guy on the skull, a cane is useful for hooking ankles (and necks), and for sharp little movements such as snapping the tip of the cane up into the opponent's genitals. This attack requires only a wrist motion and is almost impossible to anticipate or block.

Can Opener: The hand-powered kind with the sharp tine on the end. Excellent for striking into the eyes and face.

Car: The use of an automobile as a moving weapon is common in TV gangster movies. If the gangsters try to pull you over on the street you can use the same approach. If they are in a car you can sideswipe them and run them off the road. If they are on foot . . . .

Car Door: A car door presents possibilities similar to a cabinet door. If you are in the car you can thrust the door open violently with your feet, hitting your attacker in the shins. If you

50

are the party on the sidewalk, let the adversary open the door and put one foot on the pavement. Then kick the door shut again. (See Figure 20.)

Car Window Handle: If you are abducted and thrown in the back seat of a car you may find that your captors have thoughtfully removed the door handles to hinder your efforts at escape. The window cranks may still be there, however. If you get the opportunity, you may feel the urge to pull the window handle free from the door and drive it solidly into the driver's head

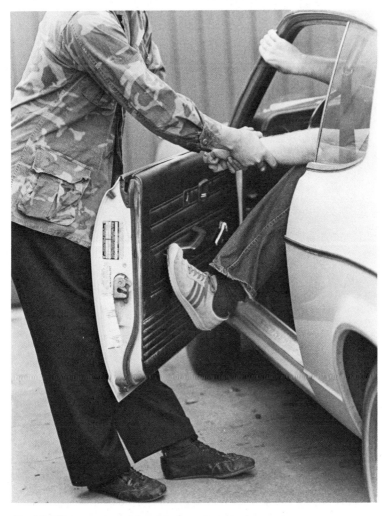

Fig. 20: When an angry driver tries to pull you from your car, use the door for a crippling opening move.

about an inch in front of his ear.

Cartridges: In those thrilling days of yesteryear the Lone Ranger used to toss a few .44 cartridges into the rustlers' fire to create a diversion. Some of the larger rifle cartridges are big enough to be used like daggers to stab at the eyes and throat. Three inch magnum shotshells are heavy enough to use as bludgeons when clenched in the fist. (Be sure to hit with the

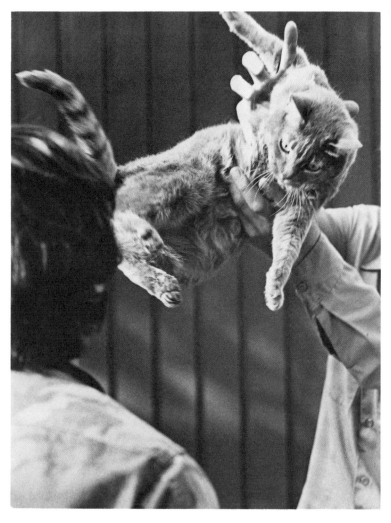

Fig. 21: **We do not normally think of a cat as an ally in a fight, but a cat as a projectile can be a ferocious thing. Aim tabby at the opponent's face and follow through with a kick to his groin.**

crimped end . . . not the primer!)

Casement Window: Slam it shut on the opponent's head or hand. This might not sound too easy because of the difficulty of getting him to oblige by sticking his head in the window, right? Well, what if the opponent is a burglar trying to crawl in? Slam!

Cat: Have you ever had some inconsiderate person throw a frightened cat at your face? Twenty needle-sharp claws all try to fasten themselves in your skin at once. Even the most battle-hardened warrior is put off his stride by this attack. (See Figure 21.)

CB Microphone: Hold it by the plug and swing the mike like a flail or mace-and-chain. Alternately, you can use the cord as a garrote or to secure a prisoner. But try out the radio first. You might be able to call for help. (See Figure 22.)

Chain: Such as a six-foot length of 3/8 inch case-hardened chain for locking up a bicycle. It takes two hands to swing it, and when it hits, every link does damage. It is a little-known fact that when a chain wraps itself around someone's head the free end moves faster and faster as it becomes shorter. Those last few heavy links *really* have an impact.

Chainsaw: Chainsaws are dangerous even when used just for cutting wood. A running chainsaw is a weapon no one can stand up to without a gun. Even the noise has an intimidating effect. A chainsaw isn't quite as effective when it is turned off, but in desperate hands it can still inflict some very ugly wounds. Lastly, by removing the chain itself, you can arm yourself with what amounts to a toothy bicycle chain. (See Figure 23.)

Chair: A chair is a very formidable weapon. Use the wooden straight-back variety and hold it lion-tamer fashion. Thrust the four feet of the chair at the opponent, trying to hit him simultaneously in the groin and solar plexus, or the solar plexus and throat. No matter which leg he avoids, one of the others will get through and hurt him. If you are defending against a knife attack, the seat of the chair forms a shield while the legs press the counterattack. In the movies you always see someone getting hit over the head with a chair. Don't try it. Such an attack is too slow and leaves you wide open for a pre-emptive punch, kick or stab in the body while your arms are holding the chair over your head.

Cigarette: A lighted cigarette isn't of much use for striking powerful blows, and it can't accomplish much in terms of serious burns, either. It *can* provide an excellent distraction prior to an attack, however. There are three possibilities. Drop the lighted cigarette in a waste paper basket in front of one of your captors. There will be a split second when he will be staring at the waste basket instead of at you. Hit him then. Second, you can try something as simple as blowing smoke into his eyes, then attack as he jerks his head away. Third, with a little luck you can drop the lighted cigarette down the back of the guard's neck (or even another prisoner's neck) and make mischief during the confusion.

Cigarette Lighter: The electric cigarette lighter in a car can be heated red-hot and casually applied to an unwanted passenger like a branding iron. Not only does it repulse him but it marks him, too. A pocket lighter is obviously a source of fire, and can also be the source of a blinding spray of fuel.

Cleanser: A handful of powdered tub-and-tile cleaner thrown in the opponent's face will assault his eyes, nose and lungs. Be careful not to breathe any yourself.

Cleaver: This eldritch device will take off fingers and split skulls if necessary. There's one in almost every kitchen.

Clothesline: Need a few feet of strong cord to tie up the bad guys, make a garrote, or tie ankle-high across the top of a dark stairway? Look in the backyard.

Coat: A coat or a jacket can be stretched tightly between two clenched fists and used as a shield against a knife, club or chain attack.

Coffee Cup: A hard plastic or ceramic teacup looks perfectly innocent in the hands of a kidnap victim. When grasped with the palm over the top of the cup, the narrow bottom can be used to strike a very satisfying blow for freedom. Aim at the temple or solar plexus.

Coins: What is a robber going to ask you for? Money. So pull out a handful of bills and change and let a few coins fall to the pavement in the process. It takes superhuman control not to glance down at the bouncing coins for a second. That's when you toss the rest of the money in his face and punt his groin into next week.

Comb: Any kind of comb will do, but a steel or aluminum rat-tail comb is best. Use the teeth to slash saw-like at the opponent's face and hands. The sharply pointed handle of a rat-tail comb is excellent for stabbing at the throat, face and eyes. (See Figure 24.)

Crowbar: A crowbar is a lethal club, and the hook can be used as a penetrating edge which swung like a tomahawk.

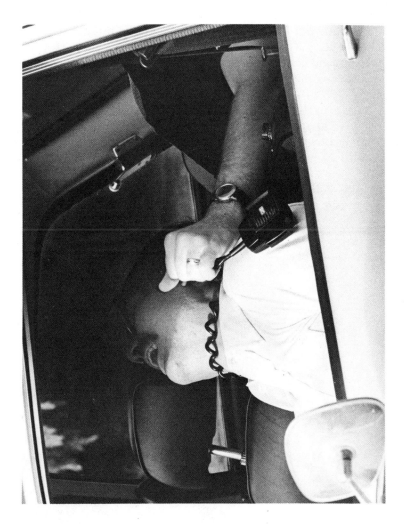

Fig. 22: A radio microphone can be used as a garrote or a mace-and-chain.

Curtain Rod: Check to see what holds up the window curtains. If it is a sturdy metal curtain rod you can use it for thrusting at the solar plexus or groin. You can also whip it across the opponent's face or snap it up into his testicles (see *cane*).

Darts: Toy darts can be thrown at an attacker's eyes, or clenched in your fist and driven into the side of his head with a hammer blow.

Deodorant Spray: Ever get any in your eyes or mouth? It's

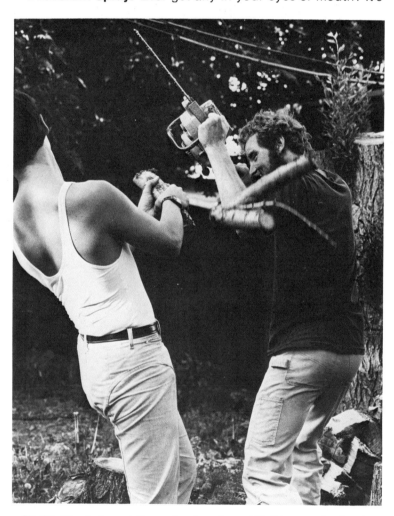

Fig. 23: The chainsaw is the modern broadsword. Nothing can stand against it except a gun.

awful. If you are cornered in the bathroom by an intruder, deodorize him . . .face first.

Dirt: The old handful-of-dirt-in-the-eyes trick.

Diving Knife: A scuba diving knife is usually an oversized bowie or dagger design with a hammer-like pommel. Of course you can chop, stab and slash with such a knife, but you can also deliver skull-shattering blows with the pommel.

Dog: A loyal dog can be a surprising help in a fight. Even if not attack-trained, your quiet little shepherd may bare her teeth and charge if someone strikes you. I saw it happen under perfectly innocent circumstances. A guest choked on a bite of food, and her husband started to slap her on the back to help her. He landed one slap and the gentlest dog I ever met sank her teeth into his wrist and wouldn't let go. Of course, if you have a toy poodle it might be best to just grab it by the hind legs and use it as a club.

Door: As your kidnapper motions you into the next room, turn and slam the door into his face. Or, if someone tries to force his way into your apartment, slam the door on his leg or gun hand. (See Figure 25.)

Drain Cleaner: This is extremely caustic when thrown into an opponent's eyes, nose or mouth. A solution of drain cleaner and water is even more effective because it burns the skin, too.

Drain Stopper: A bathtub plug with a chain. Detach it from the tub and use it as a flail. It will work better if you can slip some big steel washers on the chain, or gouge a hole through a bar of soap and slip it on to the chain first.

Drawer: A drawer can be kicked shut on the adversary's hand, pulled out and dropped on his foot, dumped on the floor for a distraction, or flung frisbee-like across the room at the opponent's head.

Drinking Glass: Toss the water in his eyes and hit him with the thick glass base. Strike for the bridge of the nose, the teeth, the side of the jaw or the temple. Or you can hold the glass by the base, shatter the top, and slash with it.

Enema Syringe: Give him a shot of hot water or rubbing alcohol, and then ram the syringe about three inches into his ear canal.

Extension Cord: Use as a garrote, a noose, a trip-cord, or to bind the hands and feet of a prisoner. You can also plug it into a wall and use it to electrify a door handle or some similar object which the kidnapper is likely to touch.

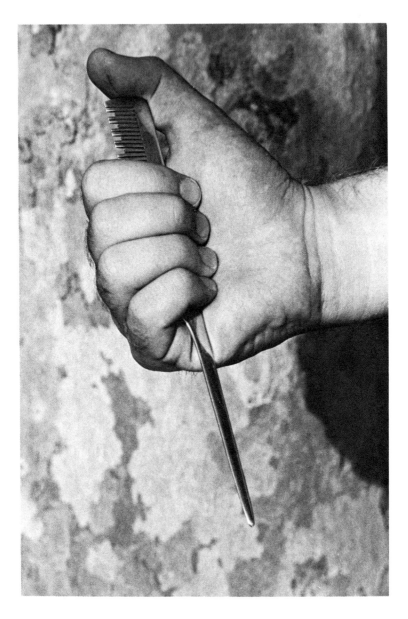

Fig. 24: A steel, rat-tail comb is perfectly legal to carry. The pointed handle and the saw-like teeth can do severe damage in the right hands.

Eyeglasses: Fold the stems in against the lenses and grasp the whole apparatus in your fist. Strike hammer-like blows with the sharp hinged corner between the frame and the stem. If you have time, crush the lenses and throw the glass fragments into the opponent's eyes before striking.

Face Towel: Fold the corners together to form a bag. Drop a new bar of soap into the bag and twist the towel to make a

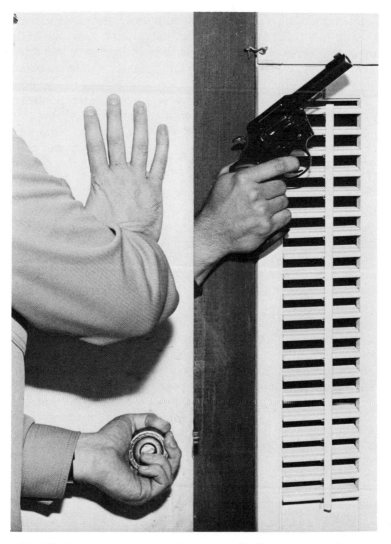

Fig. 25: **Even a front door can be a very effective weapon under some circumstances.**

simple blackjack. (See Figure 15.)

Faggot: A flaming bundle of wood or a flaming stick. A club is an effective and intimidating weapon. When it is *on fire* it is even more intimidating. Thrust the burning end of the stick at his face and let him bat at it with his hands. Get it caught in his clothing if possible.

Filleting Knife: All you fishermen take note. A typical filleting knife has a very long, narrow and thin blade which looks like it ought to be really good for stabbing. Unfortunately, such a blade is too flimsy for heavy thrusts. It can easily bend or break and leave you defenseless. It is far better to use it for slashing only. Slash at the opponent's hands, wrists, face and neck for best effect.

Fire: The potential for fire as a weapon or a distraction is so great that we will return to it again and again in this list (for instance, see *candle* and *faggot*). Anytime you see fire in any form it represents an opportunity to injure or panic your captors. People have a natural fear of fire . . . with good reason when it is used as a weapon. (See Figure 26.)

Fire Extinguisher: A pressurized fire extinguisher is designed to be snatched from its wall bracket and discharged easily. Discharge it in the kidnapper's face or use it to fill the room with clouds of dust and vapor as a smokescreen. Then hit him over the head with the heavy metal pressure bottle. For a more unusual application, stick a pencil or other sharp rod down the discharge tube of a CO_2 fire extinguisher. Voila! A speargun!

Fishing Line: Heavy monofilament nylon fishing line is nearly invisible. It's the perfect material for a trip cord stretched between a table and chair, or tied across the top of a staircase.

Fishing Rod: There is an authenticated case of a fisherman holding off an attacking grizzly bear by jabbing the tip of his rod in the bear's eyes. Against a person you can jab with the rod's tip or whip it (line guides and all) across his face.

Fishing Sinker: A large fishing sinker is deadly when swung at the end of a length of cord.

Flashlight: A 5-cell flashlight is a heavy, convenient club which produces enough light to blind an opponent temporarily as you attack. If you have to walk down a dark street sometime take your flashlight with you. No district attorney would press charges against you for carrying a flashlight at night, even if you kill a mugger with it. In the daytime, however . . . .

Flashlight Battery: A single D-cell is big enough, heavy

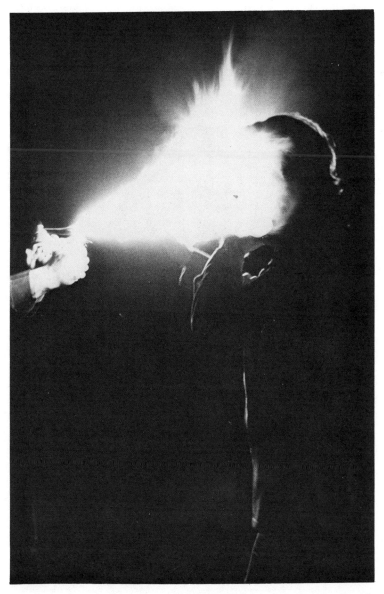

Fig. 26: Fire is a terrifying makeshift weapon. Here a disposable cigarette lighter and a can of spray lubricant are combined to create a makeshift flame-thrower.

enough, and hard enough to use for throwing or hammering on an opponent's head or collarbone.

Folding Chair: A folding chair is used to block a knife attack just like a straight-back chair (see *chair*) with the significant exception that when you block a thrust with a folding chair you can clamp the attacker's arm by collapsing the chair on it.

Fork: A table fork is hard and sharp enough to give you a tiny edge in a fight.

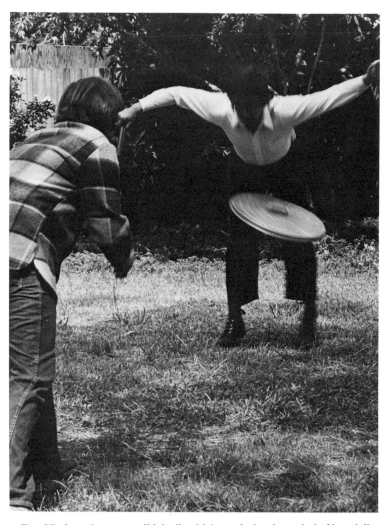

Fig. 27: A garbage can lid is the frisbee of street combat. Aim at the attacker's shins.

Garbage Can Lid: Obviously useful as a shield, a garbage can lid can also be held by the edge for battering or thrown like a frisbee into a pursuer's shins. (See Figure 27.)

Gasoline: Suppose you are incarcerated in an abandoned garage, where you happen to find half a gallon of gas in an old can. Imagine the consternation of your kidnapper when you douse him with the fuel and *dare* him to shoot at you as you walk out!

Glass: As in windows. A sliver of broken glass is the sharpest edge known to science. Shatter a window, a glass cabinet door or a glass table and select a good sharp "blade." Don't pick one that is too narrow. A piece about three inches wide which tapers to a point is best. Wrap the "hilt" of your knife in cloth, such as a pillowcase or undershirt. Stab upward under the jaw. (See Figure 28.)

Gloves: A glove can be filled with rocks, change, sand, birdshot or any similar substance and used as a makeshift blackjack. Gloves are also very useful in terms of handling scalding hot pans, flaming sticks, live electrical wiring, and broken glass. And if you smash your knuckles into the other guy's teeth, the gloves will see to it that you don't cut your skin.

Golf Club: It's obviously a club, good for rapping on someone's head. It is also an excellent *cane* (see above) which can be reversed to use the handle as a whip or flail.

Guitar: The resemblance of a guitar to a baseball bat is too obvious to require much comment here. Offer to play a tune. Maybe he'll hear birdies while he is seeing stars.

Guitar String: Most guitar strings come with a little metal bead woven into the bridge end of the string. Pass the free end through the center of the bead and you have one of the simplest and strongest garrote nooses known. Tie the loose end around something you can use as a handle, such as a pen or a piece of silverware.

Hairbrush: The stiff bristles are painful when raked across the face and eyes. The side of a flat-backed brush can be used for striking blows at an opponent's neck and temple. The end of the handle is good for hammer blows against his skull, collarbone and ribs. If some character insists on bothering you, teach him a new meaning of "the brush off."

Hairspray: A woman can carry a small pressurized can of hair spray in her purse without exciting comment, right? Many brands are just as effective as tear gas when sprayed in an attacker's eyes and mouth. (See *deodorant spray*.)

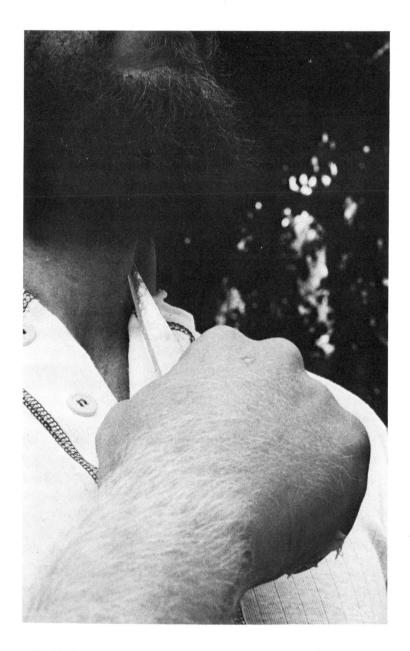

Fig. 28: Broken from a window, mirror or picture frame, a shard of glass has the sharpest cutting edge known to man. Wrap the "hilt" in a scrap of cloth to protect your hand.

Hammer: The utility of a hammer as a short war club is obvious to everyone. For added psychological effect, hold the hammer with the claws forward. That way you get a cutting effect as well as a powerful blow.

Hard Hat: Hold it in both hands as a shield, or hold it by the rim and strike with the visor edge.

Hatchet: A small hatchet can be swung like an axe or used as a club. Always be ready to "bury the hatchet" . . . the head of the hatchet, that is. (See Figure 29.)

Hat Pin: The main defensive armament of little old ladies everywhere. A hat pin is of limited utility for defense because it is so likely to bend during the first stab. It can be put to good use against the eyes, the eardrums, or when jabbed up under the jaw into the base of the tongue, however. There is also a legendary assassination technique which involves a hatpin inserted into the brain through the brain stem. The technique is rumored to be almost impossible to detect, but has little application to the context of hand-to-hand combat.

Helmet: As in motorcyle. Swing it by the chin strap.

Hoe: Although you might be inclined to chop with the blade, it is better to lunge with the handle. Drive it deep into the bad guy's throat or stomach.

Hose: A garden water hose will temporarily blind an assailant if you spray water in his face. Then grasp the hose about two feet from the end and crack him on the head with the nozzle. Alternately, a two foot length of rubber hose used as a club or flail produces the most excruciating kind of pain without breaking any bones.

Hubcap: Assaulted while changing a flat tire? It could happen in the wrong neighborhood. Use the hubcap as a shield or strike at the attackers with the edge. You can also hook your fingers inside the hubcap and smash it flat against the opponent's face or skull. Lead off by using the hubcap to scoop dirt into the attacker's eyes.

Icepick: This is another case where the weapon can be found in most kitchens, and in not a few workshops. Stab at the eyes and throat, or hammer with the butt of the handle. Stabbing to the chest is not likely to stop the attacker's onslaught until too late. One diabolical application is to casually pick up the icepick and nail the opponent's hand to the table as an opening gambit.

Iron: A hot electric iron can be used as a shield with special success because an opponent can't easily grab it away from you. Use the point for blows to the head, or swing it by the power cord for maximum damage.

Jack Handle: Another convenient weapon when changing a tire on a dark and lonely road.

Kerosene Lamp: Shatter the lip of the chimney and slash with it like a broken bottle. Pour the kerosene in a cup and splash it in your abductor's face. The glass base of a kerosene lamp is hard, heavy and easy to grip. Use it as a bludgeon. Lastly, you can smash the lighted lamp against the wall or floor and burn away the darkness.

Keys: A ring of keys can be dropped as a distraction, thrown in the attacker's face, or used as makeshift brass knuckles. For the latter, hold the key ring in the palm of your hand with keys protruding between your fingers. Strike for the nerve pressure points in the face and neck (see **Black Medicine Vol. I** for a description of a dozen such targets).

Key Chain: The reference here is to a key ring attached to a retractable chain attached to the belt. A perfectly legal device to have on one's person at all times. Unclip the chain from the belt and swing the keys like a mace-and-chain.

Kitchen Knife: It's amazing how many unarmed Americans die without a fight when every kitchen in the country is liberally stocked with deadly weapons. Grab a butcher knife or boning knife from the kitchen drawer as the intruder is coming down the hall. Hold it point down in your fist, with the edge facing forward. Hide it behind your back. When he gets close enough, whip it out and across his throat before he knows what has happened. Go for the carotid artery, and get a real slice of life. (See Figure 30.)

Knitting Needle: Many ladies carry a bag of knitting with them everywhere. What could be more natural than to include one or two especially large, sharp needles in the bag? If assaulted, hold one needle in each hand and make like a porcupine. Jab at the face, hands and body. If the needles are thick enough you can use them to whip the attacker across the face and hands, too.

Lamp: A typical electric lamp with a shade, found in most living rooms. Rip off the lamp shade and confront the intruder with the bare bulb, held like a bayonet. Thrust the hot, bright bulb in his face. If the bulb gets broken, so much the better. Then you can thrust the bare electrodes at him! Just don't wander too far from that electrical outlet.

Letter Opener: Suppose you come home early and find your

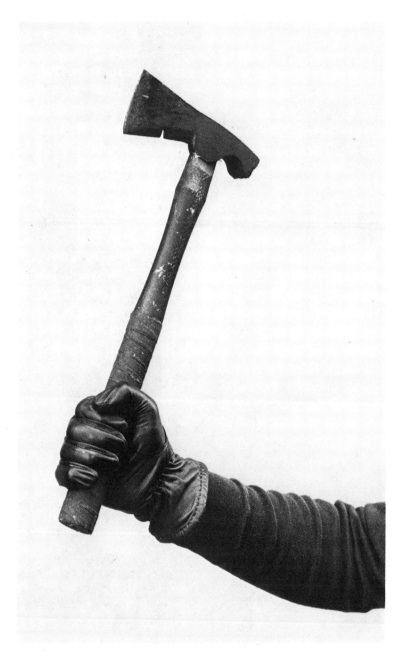

Fig. 29: **A hatchet is a tool whose potential as a weapon needs no explanation.**

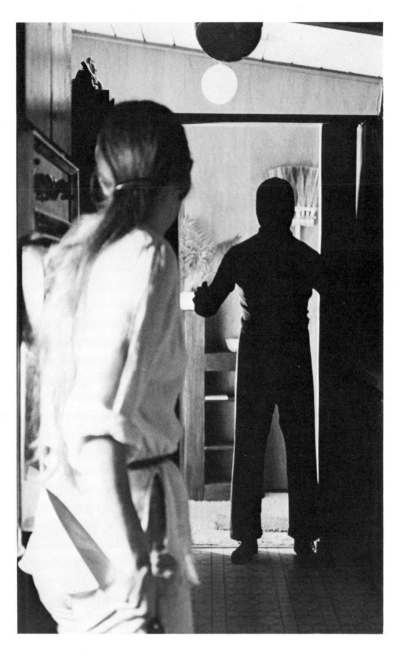

Fig. 30: When there is an intruder in the house, a kitchen knife concealed artfully behind the back could make all the difference.

wife in the arms of another man? This handy item will help you open her male.

Light Bulb: First see *lamp*, above. A light bulb clasped in the hand isn't too menacing until you hit somebody with it. Grip the base and smash the glass bulb into the side of the opponent's face. It will shatter, and in shattering it will slash dozens of cuts.

Lug Wrench: The "X" shaped kind are great for throwing, especially at the legs of an assailant in close pursuit.

Magazine: Roll it up into a tight baton, then stab and hammer with the ends. You can swat with it but the effect is minimal except against eardrums (and flies). If the magazine is too small to be effective, roll it up tightly and then bend it in half. The folded end is amazingly solid.

Matchbox: In Fairbairn's combat text **Get Tough!** there is an amusing suggestion that you can kill an enemy soldier by whacking him in the side of the head with a 2" box of wooden matches. Fairbairn says to clench the matchbox in your fist and strike a hammer-like blow on the soldier's temple. The blow could easily kill the soldier, but it is the *fist*, not the matchbox, which does the damage. This illustrates a very important point about certain makeshift weapons. In many cases the real function of the "weapon" is to convince you that you are not hitting the enemy with your bare hand. If you believe that you are striking with some object (no matter how puny) you lose your fear of hurting your hand. As a result you hit a lot harder. Karate artists train for many months before learning to suppress their fear of self-injury, which then allows them to split boards, crack stones, break bricks and crush skulls with their bare hands. You can make this powerful advantage work for you simply by holding *anything* in your hand while you strike. Even a matchbox. It really works.

Mirror: A large mirror is raw material for a glass dagger (see *glass*). A smaller face mirror with a handle is a pretty good club. Use the narrow edge like a hatchet on the opponent's wrists and face.

Mouthwash: Slosh it or spit it into the opponent's eyes. Then hit him with the bottle.

Newspaper: Best when rolled into a tight cylinder about 15 inches long and 2 inches in diameter. A rolled newspaper is effective for swatting at incoming punches and knife attacks, but its real strength lies in jabs with the end of the roll. The end of a tightly rolled newspaper is very hard and strong. It makes a big impression when jabbed stiffly into someone's groin, solar plexus, throat or eye. For variety, you can smack him over the ear with it and break his eardrum.

Notebook: The blue, canvas-covered 3-ring binder favored by high school and college students. Held with two hands it can be used as a shield to fend off fist, knife and club attacks. From the same position you can counterattack by ramming the spine of the notebook up under the attacker's chin or nose. One-handed, the notebook can be swung like an axe at the face, forearms, or side of the neck. Turned inside-out, the open half-rings of the binder form formidable claws when jammed into an attacker's face.

Onion: Der gas warfare! Under the right circumstances a hot onion could provide an opening for an attack against your kidnappers or guards. A handful of minced onion forcefully applied to the face can blind and choke the victim temporarily. (At least long enough for you to blind or choke him permanently.)

Oven Cleaner: Especially the spray kind. Extremely caustic. Don't get any on yourself while you are spraying it on everybody else.

Paint: Once again, it's best in a spray can but an open bucket will do. Paint has all the advantages of other spray products in terms of blinding the opponent, but it also *marks* him. If you dump a bucket of orange paint on the kidnapper's head and run outside into the street, he probably won't follow. It's very difficult to remain inconspicuous when you are bright green, for instance.

Paperweight: Almost any kind of paperweight is small enough, hard enough and heavy enough to be used as a bludgeon. You can smash a skull with it, to put it bluntly.

Paring Knife: A small, short-bladed kitchen knife should be used only for slashing at the face and hands, or possibly for stabbing into the throat. The blade is not long enough or strong enough for stabbing into the abdomen and rib cage.

Pen: Held like a knife it can be used for jabbing at the eyes, throat and the nerves under the ears (see **Black Medicine Vol. I** for details). When clenched in the fist it can be driven through the cranial wall by a fist-hammer attack. For the adept, there are many nerve attacks which use the pen as a deep probe. One example would be to strike backward with the pen into the assailant's inguinal triangle when embraced from behind.

Pen Knife: A very small pocket knife. Useless as a knife, it can still serve as a weapon when wielded like a pen (see above).

Pencil: Like a pen (see above) but more pointed for deeper penetrating, and more brittle (which means less power). A pencil is best for stabbing at the eyes and the hollow of the throat. Also good for attacking the eardrum. Cannot be driven through the skull wall except occasionally at the temple.

Penlight: Almost as good as a pen for power blows (see *pen*). A penlight has the added advantage of its beam of bright light. If the fracas occurs after dark you can dazzle your opponent's vision by keeping the beam focused on his eyes. Squinting into the light he will have trouble seeing your kick coming until too late.

Pepper: What kind of brutish kidnapper wouldn't allow you some pepper for your food? Be casual. "Pass the pepper, please." Pretend there is something wrong with the shaker. Unscrew the lid and sling the contents in his face. Overturn the table in his lap or slug him with the shaker for good measure.

Picture Frame: A typical picture frame consists of four stout pieces of wood tacked together at the corners. Take the picture down from the wall and kick out the center. Smash the corner of the frame against the floor and pry off a nice club with a sharply pointed end.

Pill Bottles: The bottle itself can be clenched in the fist as a weapon, or you can dump the pills in the kidnapper's coffee. Improvise! Dump most of a bottle of aspirin down the toilet, and then claim you swallowed it. Act drowsy and increasingly uncoordinated. Then, while the kidnappers are frantically trying to revive you . . . attack.

Pillow: In the movies you always see the bad guy suffocate the helpless hospital patient with a pillow. People who have really tried it will tell you that suffocation by pillow is a long and horrible process, involving pulmonary convulsions, vomiting, and the ever-present possibility that the victim may get in a lucky punch and turn the tables on you. My advice is to use a pillow only as a shield against a fist or knife attack (see *coat*).

Pingpong Paddle: Chop with the edge of the blade, or hammer with the base of the handle. Don't swat, it doesn't work.

Pipe (Plumbing): An 18 inch length of lead pipe makes a deadly bludgeon. It's slow to swing but it does appalling damage.

Pipe (Smoking): Hold it like a pistol and jab at the eyes with the stem, or grasp the stem in your fist and hammer with the bowl. Don't overlook the possibility of casting the coal or ashes into the opponent's eyes as an opening gambit.

Pistol: Here's some advice regarding taking a pistol away from your attacker . . . don't. Unless you know exactly what you are doing, and the opponent is a total fool, such an attempt is suicidal. Then again, if it looks like you are going to die anyway, what would you have to lose? We'll assume that somehow you are engaged in hand-to-hand combat and there is a pistol in your hand. If the pistol is loaded, shoot somebody. You can see that a revolver is loaded by glancing in the front of the cylinder . . . not the barrel. In an automatic pull the slide back and look inside. Or just point it at the bad guy and pull the trigger. If it's loaded it will fire. If not you can use the pistol as a makeshift weapon three ways. Hold it normally and jab at the solar plexus, throat or eyes with the muzzle. If it's a revolver, you can hold it by the barrel and swing the butt like a hammer at the opponent's head. An automatic should be held by the slide to strike with the rear sight. (See Figure 31.)

Pitchfork: A man holding a pitchfork can be very intimidating. Just don't forget that the handle makes a more versatile weapon than the tines.

Phonograph Records: Can be thrown like a frisbee or a dinner plate, and can also be broken if you need something sharp and pointed.

Plate: A ceramic or heavy plastic dinner plate can be held to deliver vicious chopping blows with the edge. Keep this in mind when your kidnappers bring you your dinner.

Pocket Knife: The effectiveness of a pocket knife depends mainly on its size. A small knife (2½ inch blade) *can* be used for slashing, but it is better to use the body of the knife like a pen (see above) for hammer-like blows to the skull, collarbone and ribs. A larger knife with a locking 4 or 5 inch blade can be used for actual knife dueling if you are so inclined.

Poker: If there is a fireplace in the room there is probably a cast iron poker, too. Most pokers are about a foot and a half long with an iron point and a recurved hook. You can swing a poker like a club or (obviously) you can poke with it. The most vicious attack is to snap the poker up into the opponent's groin, then rip it straight out with the hook turned up.

Pool Ball: The balls on a pool table can be used like baseballs (see above) for throwing, but the fact that they are usually found in groups of a dozen or more lends them to rapid-fire throwing. Aim at the face or groin.

Pool Cue: A hardwood pool cue is an excellent lance-like

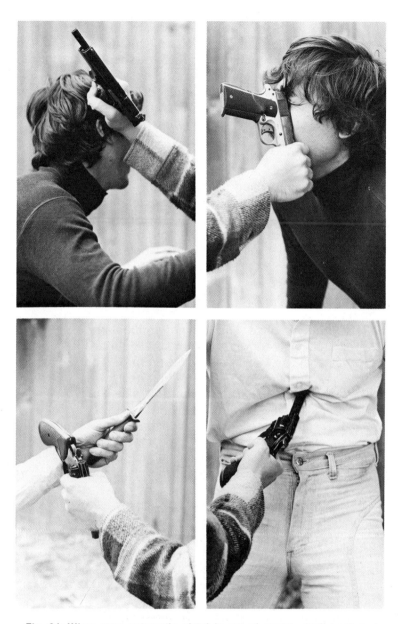

Fig. 31: When your automatic pistol is out of ammo, don't hesitate to hammer with it. A blow to the temple is especially lethal *(top left).* Striking with the pistol's rear sights intensifies the power of the blow *(top right).* The hooked shape of a revolver can be useful for catching the opponent's hand, and the butt is well-known for its hammer-like qualities *(below left).* A very effective move is to ram the pistol barrel into the opponent's solar plexus *(below right).*

staff. Hold it with the heavy end forward so you can rap it sideways as well as jab with the end. Oriental stick fighting techniques are well documented, and you should study them if you spend a lot of time in sleazy pool halls.

Powdered Soap: Powdered laundry detergent is even better than pepper as an eye and nose irritant. Throw a handful in the face of your assailant the next time you get mugged at the laundromat.

Purse: Even if you aren't in the habit of carrying a purse the odds are that someone close by will have one when trouble starts. Use it as a shield (see *notebook* and *coat*) or glance inside for a *comb, pocket knife* or *pen*.

Rake: The lighter the better. Use a rake like a *broom* to lunge and strike at the opponent's face, throat, and forearms. The teeth of the rake can be punishing when swept across the opponent's face, or they may be employed to scoop and throw a mixture of dirt and leaves into his eyes. Once again, remember to hold the rake with the handle toward the enemy. The handle is a better weapon than the teeth.

Rattail File: I once had a brief infatuation with knife-throwing, during which I discovered that a rattail file from the tool chest makes an excellent throwing spike. Throw it underhand with the sharp tang forward. At ranges of six to ten feet you can drive that tang up to an inch into a pine board. Aim for the opponent's face.

Razor Blade: A slash with a razor blade can sever tendons in the wrist, spill an impressive quantity of the opponent's blood, or even sever the carotid artery and jugular vein. Wrap a scrap of paper around the rear edge of the blade to protect your fingers while you attack.

Rifle: A rifle or shotgun is a deadly weapon even without any ammunition. As with the *pistol* the first thing to do is to bluff that the gun is loaded. Failing that, use the muzzle to drive lance-like attacks into the enemy's face and body. Follow through with smashing strokes from the butt of the piece. Don't forget that even the middle of a rifle can be used for blows up under the jaw or into the face.

Rocks: One of man's oldest weapons. Used for throwing and hammering like *baseballs, paperweights* and *pool balls.* Rocks have an added advantage of being found almost everywhere outdoors, usually associated with useful amounts of *dirt.* Use the two together for a combined diversion and attack.

Rolling Pin: The symbol of the domineering wife. Using a rolling pin as a makeshift weapon has a unique advantage. We have all seen the image of the wife beating the husband over the head so often that when you pick up a rolling pin your opponent will expect the stereotype attack. That's fine. Raise the rolling pin high in the air as if about to swing at his head. Then while he is staring at it you can kick him in the groin. If he succeeds in blocking the kick he'll have to look down first. *That's when you swing the pin!*

Rug: A small throw rug can be used like a *coat* or *bath towel* or you can try the old trick where you jerk the rug out from under the other guy's feet. It takes good timing but it can be done.

Salt: It isn't as irritating as *pepper* but it can be used in almost the same way. Another possibility is to substitute salt for sugar in the guards' sugar bowl. Be ready to move when one of them suddenly chokes on his coffee.

Safety Razor: The old-fashioned kind with the flat steel top should be gripped crosswise in the fist, the stem between the middle and ring fingers and the head forming a shield in front of the knuckles. Use like brass knuckles. Alternately, you can grip it with the head protruding from the bottom of the fist for hammer blows.

Saucer: A small *plate.* A saucer should be held edgewise for chopping to put a sharp edge on a palm-heel attack. Rest the edge of the saucer across the palm of your hand with your thumb on one side and fingers on the other. Now ram it up under the opponent's nose as hard as you can.

Saw: Any kind of handsaw. Slash with the teeth at the adversary's face, neck, and especially his hands.

Scissors: Best for jabbing. Hold the scissors locked open as far as they will go and stab with the sharply pointed blade. You can also hold the scissors normally, open them about 2 inches, and stab for the eyes.

Screwdriver: A weapon which can be found in most kitchens and all workshops. Hold it normally to stab with the bit or hammer with the base of the handle. Reverse your grip to swing the handle like a club.

Sex: Feigned sexual acquiescence to a rapist can be a powerful weapon for a young woman. I am reminded of one resourceful lady who "gave in" enthusiastically, and right in the middle of giving the rapist a good time suddenly yanked his testicles down to his knees and let them snap up again like a windowshade. She walked away unharmed.

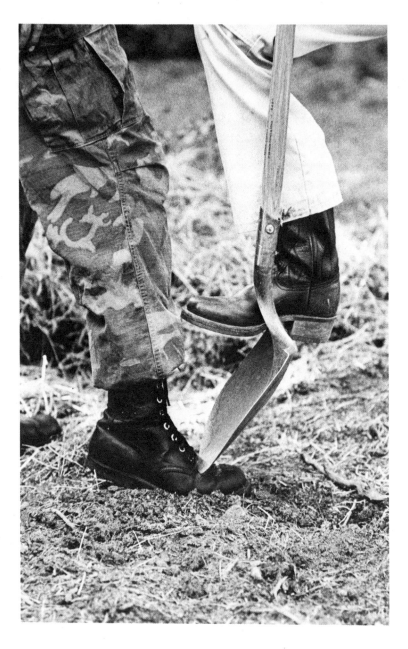

Fig. 32: "What did you say, stranger?" Even though pictured here as a cutting implement, a shovel is more versatile as a staff. While the opponent is warily watching the blade you can rap him on the head with the handle!

76

Shit: There is an old story about an oriental warrior who made a mess in his pants, let it slide down his pant leg, and then kicked it into the face of his enemy as a diversion. Just keep in mind the fact that if your place of confinement doesn't contain any dirt to throw in the kidnapper's face, you can always *make* some!

Shoes: Shoes make any kind of kick more penetrating and effective. They can also be thrown, or used as clubs or hammers. High-heeled shoes are especially effective for hammer-like blows. Ripping the heel off of a shoe gives you a convenient tiger-paw studded with short, sharp nails.

Shoestring: Use it to secure a prisoner by tying his thumbs together behind his back. If the shoestrings are strong enough you can use them to form a trip line or garrote.

Shovel: Unlike a broom or rake, a shovel has a strong cutting edge which can be used in combat. The shovel blade may be used for thrusting, sideways chopping, or blows with the flat side. Of course, it's only natural to scoop dirt in the opponent's face. For fast surprise attacks always use the handle, not the blade. The guy who is making you dig your own grave will be wary of the shovel blade, but will relax a little when you turn it away from him. That's when you ram the handle into his gut. (See Figure 32.)

Silver Dollars: Real silver dollars are heavy discs of metal which can be thrown *hard* at an opponent's face with a significant possibility of doing some damage. With a little practice you can lodge a silver dollar in a pine board (edge-on) just like a small knife. Some people carry their silver dollars in small leather drawstring bags which they hang from their belts. When swung by the drawstring this change purse becomes a formidable blackjack. And there is one big advantage. The government can't possible outlaw carrying concealed *money*, now can they?

Ski Poles: Ski poles make good substitutes for rapiers, short lances, or canes. If you pry the basket off the end you can stab deeply with them, and they are easy to use in a whipping motion. Reverse the pole and strike with the handle for more powerful sideways or downward blows. (See *cane*.)

Ski Wax: Use it like a *bar of soap* to make an improvised blackjack.

Skis: You would think that a fighter wearing skis would be fatally handicapped, but it isn't necessarily true. The length of the ski gives tremendous range and penetration to both front and back kicks. You can kick the point of the ski into an opponent's groin or abdomen as much as six or seven feet away. And the effect which the sharp outer edge of a ski has on someone's shin is devastating. If you have time to take the skis off, you can use one quarterstaff style for lunging and battering at the opponent.

Socks: Can be used as a garrote if long enough. Best employed as part of a sock-and-soap blackjack (see *bar of soap*).

Spoon: Use it to gouge at the opponent's eyes and nerve centers.

Staff: When people go hiking in the mountains they frequently carry with them a hiking staff, a length of one-inch diameter branch or pole for leaning on or for clubbing snakes. It's very good for clubbing two-legged snakes, too, and in the hands of a skilled fighter it makes a man more than a match for half a dozen unarmed antagonists. No wonder the ancient Chinese monks carried them everywhere.

Stairway: If you are being escorted up a stairway pretend to trip on the risers. Catch yourself on your hands and kick viciously backward into the guard's groin or knees. Make him fall backward down the stairs, then leap down on him heels first. If you are being herded *down* the stairs, suddenly drop down on your heels and jerk the guard's feet out from under him. Lift them high enough to see that he catches some steps in the back of the head.

Stool: A small stool is used as a shield (see *chair*) or as a club. It is also possible to sling a stool along the ground into the opponent's legs.

Swimming Pool: Throw a body block and spill your guard into the pool. If he fires his gun with the barrel full of water he'll regret it. Deeply.

Table Knife: Unless it is a steak knife it won't be of much use for slashing or stabbing. The best approach is to use the base of the handle for striking hammer blows to the temple and collarbone.

Telephone: If you have the opportunity, call for help. If your captors force you to talk over the phone during ransom negotiations, use the handset as a club and brain one of them. You can also throw the body of the phone at an opponent, or whirl it like a bola, entangling the enemy in the cord.

Tennis Racket: Strike chopping blows with the edge, or jam the base of the handle into the attacker's abdomen or throat.

Toilet Brush: This innocuous item is found in most bathrooms, usually residing in a small pail beside the toilet. The end of the handle offers the usual potential for hammer blows, and the brush end is very effective when jammed into the eyes. For added effect, bu sure that you smear the brush in something really repulsive first. (See *shit*.)

Toilet Paper: I wish that I could tell you to smack somebody in the side of the head with a roll of TP to kill him, but it just doesn't work too well. The roll of cardboard in the center, though, does have possibilities. Extract it from the tissue and roll it into a tight, hard cylinder. Use it like a pen to hammer at his face and temple. Then there is the "spit-wad" attack, in which you soak a fist-sized wad of TP in bleach and smack it into the opponent's eyes.

Toothbrush: What could be a more natural thing to demand from your kidnappers than to be allowed to brush your teeth? No harm in that, right? When the guards aren't looking, stroke the bristles across a bar of wet soap. Then use your thumb to flick the bristles into a guard's face, spraying soap droplets into his eyes. When he grabs his eyes ram the brush as far up his nose as it will go (or into his ear).

Umbrella: The best kind has a heavy wooden handle and a steel spike on the end. When closed an umbrella is used like a *cane* for slashing and jabbing at the throat, solar plexus and face. When open it takes only a small movement to ram the ends of the stays into the opponent's eyes.

Urine: Many pieces of light cloth (such as a T-shirt) are ineffective weapons when dry, but make formidable flails when wet. Use some of nature's fountain and get to work!

Wash Cloth: Dripping with scalding hot, soapy water. Throw it into the guard's face, then follow through with a kick in a tender spot.

Watch: Many people say that the band of a watch can be slipped over the knuckles to make a punch more punishing. In my experience this only works with leather bands. Otherwise the punishment is to your hand.

Windowshade Roller: An excellent, weighted club that is nearly always overlooked when clearing a room of possible weapons. Take it down off its brackets, strip off the paper shade, and use the roller for jabbing or for powerful swinging blows to the head and body. Let the sunshine in!

Wrench: One of the most effective of all small makeshift clubs. Be careful, though. A steel wrench is so heavy and so narrow that it is possible to splatter someone's head with it when you only intended to tap him.

Yo-Yo: The lowly yo-yo was originally a hand weapon, something like a cross between a bola and a boomerang. You can throw it, swing it, hammer with it, or use the string as a trip wire or garrote.